IN-SEASON TRAINING

FOR SPORT

By

Jason Shea, M.S.

IN-SEASON TRAINING

FOR SPORT

By

Jason Shea, M.S.

Table of Contents

Chapter I: Performance Deterioration   Page 1

Chapter II: In-Season Strength   Page 11

Chapter III: In-Season Weight Maintenance   Page 21

Chapter IV: In-Season Power   Page 29

Chapter V: In-Season Functional Strength   Page 43

Chapter VI: In-Season Nutrition   Page 55

Chapter VII: In-Season Injury Management   Page 69

Chapter VIII: In-Season Game Day Tips   Page 79

Chapter IX: In-Season Programming For Sport   Page 91

     In-Season Football Programming   Page 93
     In-Season Soccer Programming   Page 101
     In-Season Baseball Programming   Page 107
     In-Season Hockey Programming   Page 113
     In-Season Basketball Programming   Page 121
     In-Season Field Hockey Programming   Page 127
     In-Season Lacrosse Programming   Page 133
     In-Season Rugby Programming   Page 137
     In-Season Softball Programming   Page 143
     In-Season Golf Programming   Page 149
     In-Season Tennis Programming   Page 153
     In-Season Volleyball Programming   Page 159
     In-Season Wrestling Programming   Page 165

Chapter X: Exercise Technique   Page 171

Acknowledgements

Sitting here in front of my computer, one would think that after five plus years of collecting information, reading studies, articles, and books, interviewing experts, and of course, writing, the acknowledgements section would come easy. Truth be told; the writer's block and associated anxiety are similar to trying to formulate the opening paragraph years ago. I am not sure if it is the pressure expressing my gratitude on paper or if it is the anxiety associated with project completion. Perhaps a little of both! With that said, the following is my attempt at acknowledging anybody and everybody whom has helped, believed, and inspired me through the years in making this project finally become a reality.

First off, I would like to deeply thank Charles Poliquin for his time, infinite wisdom, and tremendous support in this project. As an old Japanese proverb states "better than a thousand days of diligent study is one day with a great teacher." Thank you for the opportunities you have provided me and the incredible doors you have opened for both me and my family. Much of what I know and do as a strength coach can be attributed what you have taught me and the people you have introduced me to. Sincerely, thank you Coach!

Next I would like to thank my incredible staff and clientele at APECS for their never-ending loyalty, dedication, and incredible support. Words cannot express the gratitude I have for you guys in giving me the constant nudge make this project become a reality.

Next a special thanks to two very important people, Jeff Dufficy and Tony Sirianni, who have helped pick me up when knocked down, taught me how to stay positive through all adversity, and inspired me to achieve better in life. I cannot thank either of you enough, nor are there enough words to describe what your never ending inspiration has meant to me. Your mentorship and friendships have been an invaluable part in me becoming the person and professional I am today. Thank you for constantly inspiring me to be better and never letting me give up on my dreams.

As there a probably too many to mention, I would like to reach out and thank a few friends and professional colleagues for their influence in the development of this book: Jay B for the constant nudges to be better as both a person and professional. Brad Sidwell for your never ending loyalty, support, and belief in what I am doing. Dr. Erin Thomas for believing in me and giving me the opportunity to teach what I have learned to others. Coaches Jon Jackson, Todd Vasey, Dan McClean, Al Necchi, Rita Atkinson, Chris Spillane, Carrie Lovoncallo, Chris Schmidt, Chris Baker, and many more for your continued support over the years. Thank you to subject matter experts, Chad Robertson, Dr. Stuart McGill, Istvan Javorek, Denis Reno, Dr. Jeff Volek, Ann and Chris Fredericks, Dr. Mark Houston, Laurie Warren, and Dr. Jonny Bowden, for giving of your valuable time and allowing me to pick your brains for the best information possible in your given fields. Thank you to Kim Goss and Nancy Olesin for your incredible professional guidance through the editorial processes. Thank you to my undergrad advisor Dr. Frank Rife for inspiring me to complete my undergrad degree and eventually earn my masters.

A special thanks to my brother Jeremy for helping me to gather all the pertinent research and studies necessary to provide a quality product. Another special thanks to my good friend Paul DiPillo for your never-ending support and help in making this project a reality.

Another special thank you to my Aunt Carol, Uncle David, Luc, Lacie, and Mac for your unbelievable support, inspiration, and for always being there when we needed you☺

An extra special thank you to my parents for constantly believing in me throughout my life and teaching me to walk tall, be strong and persevere through any challenges. You have given me both root and wings!

Lastly, I would like to give another extra special thank you to my family Ayden, Bryn, and Wendy. Thank you for your support and understanding when "Daddy" was away working all those weekends to get this done. Ayden and Bryn you are the lights of my life. Wendy, you have been my inspiration since the day we met.

Thank you all.

Sincerely,

Jason

CHAPTER I

PERFORMANCE DETERIORATION

Strength and conditioning has become an integral component of competitive sports in the modern era. Athletes spend considerable time and energy during the off-season correcting imbalances, rehabilitating injuries, and increasing strength, size, power and speed. In addition to these physical characteristics, athletes also enlist the expertise of technical and strategic coaches to improve upon skill development. All of this requires a tremendous investment of time, money, and resources in preparation for the upcoming sports season.

The result of all the hard work becomes clearly visible during tryouts and pre-season practices. With improvements in muscular coordination, speed, power, and overall athletic ability, athletes may stand out in the eyes of their coaches. The potential for success on the field has been enhanced greatly.

If athletes fail to continue with those training protocols in which these results were forged, they may fall prey to the negative effects of performance deterioration. This begs the question "what good is it to be your physical best at the beginning of season if you allow your hard earned results to rapidly deteriorate as the season progresses"?

Many athletes are under the impression they can maintain those hard-earned off-season results through the physical labors of team practice. This dramatic oversight can leave the door open for a number of negative consequences including decreases in strength, speed and power as well as increased potential for injury.

Performance deterioration, also known as detraining, reversibility, or de-adaptation, is the result of an extended period of time away from training. Quite simply, if you stop training, your hard earned results will slowly deteriorate. The body adapts to the stresses placed upon it. If the physical stresses are minimal, the resulting physical adaptations can be less than optimal. According to a 2002 study on recreationally strength trained men subjected to 3 weeks of training cessation, the researchers found "physiological changes corresponding to decreased performance capacity [17]". The extent to which the subjects' performance was decreased depended on the synergistic effects of a number of variables including training age, methodologies of training they incorporated into their regimens, and the length of cessation (17). A separate study on football players and powerlifters had similar findings (15).

Knowledge of the negative effects of de-training is important, but this is only half the picture. Coaches and athletes also need to gain an understanding of the positive effects in-season training can have on performance.

> # Did you know that with 2 training days a week during season, athletes can still lose strength?

In 1998, a group of researchers set out to test the performance and strength capabilities of football players after a season that consisted of 2 training days per week. The battery of research tests included bench press, flexibility, vertical jump, broad jump, and agility run (27). The comparative results are below:

Test Type	Pre-Season	Pre-Season	Post- Season	Post- Season
	Lineman	Non-Lineman	Lineman	Non-Lineman
Bench Press (lbs)	313.21	298.29	288.91	279.14
Flexibility (cm)	25.63	32.89	27.31	31.91
Vertical Jump (cm)	55.44	64.97	53.88	62.01
Long Jump (m)	2.39	2.61	2.38	2.58
Agility Run	4.69	4.35	4.64	4.34

Schnieder, V, Arnold, B, Martin, K, Bell, D, Crocker, P. **Detraining Effects in College Football Players During the Competitive Season.** *Journal of Strength and Conditioning Research.* 12(1); Pp 42-45. 1998.

Even with two day a-week in-season strength training, a drop in bench press strength occurred in both groups. The vertical jump and broad jump, which are predictors of total body power, also saw decreases in both groups throughout the season. On a positive note, the agility run did see a slight increase in performance for both groups.

These on-field markers used in this study, vertical jump, broad jump, and agility run, are three performance predictors used by collegiate and professional scouting combines. In fact, many athletes have been drafted and signed to multi-million dollar contracts with the aid of outstanding performances in these markers at the NFL combine. With a decrease in any of these on-field markers, an athlete may see a drop in on-field performance.

AVOIDING PERFORMANCE DETERIORIATION = MAINTAINING STRENGTH

Understanding that coaches need time to work on skill development, strategy, and conditioning during in-season practices, time should also be allotted for quick in-season strength sessions, with the objective being the team's readiness on game day.

In-season strength and conditioning should focus on gaining or at the very least maintaining strength. According to early Soviet research, "strength exercises are used more during the preparatory training period and relatively less during the competitive period. However, **specific strength exercises, which often require maximum exertion, continue to be used during the competitive period, not just to maintain strength, but also to increase strength** (13)."

Strength, power, and fitness levels need to be maintained throughout the season to avoid performance deterioration and injury, especially when competing at high levels. If an athlete attains a high level of fitness and is not required to engage in activities that will maintain that level of fitness, the potential for injury may increase.

According to former Canadian strength coach Charlie Francis, "strength is the easiest quality to build, but it is also the easiest one to lose [7]." In the past, the popular method of in-season training entailed cutting back on the intensity of training while maintaining a similar volume. For instance, if an athlete's 1Rep Max back squat was 350lbs heading into the season, then, according to this theory, a trainee would only need to perform sets of about 210lbs (60%1RM) for higher reps during their season to maintain performance. This is typically referred to as maintenance work.

The problem with this method is that athletes may be teaching their bodies to become weaker. In order to maintain or gain strength, an athlete needs to train at loads near or above 80% in order to stimulate the nervous system to recruit high threshold muscle fibers [2,3]. Maintenance training at 60% of one's max does not accomplish this.

In 2003 researchers set out to test the credibility of the 80% sub-maximal load theory by studying the strength changes of 53 NCAA Div III football players during an in-season training program. The research team found greater strength improvements in the athletes training at or above 80% 1RM when compared to those athletes using less resistance [12].

One of the major concerns coaches and athletes have with training at such high intensities during season is the possibility of disrupting the balance between proper recovery and adaptation to training stimulus. The simple solution to this problem is to cut back on volume and maintain/increase intensity.

For years, strength pioneers including world renowned strength coach Charles Poliquin, have advocated decreased volume while maintaining intensity during the competitive season [14]. Cutting the in-season training volume by 50% or more will aid in recovery whilst allowing for proper stimulation.

In simplified terms, rather than cutting back on the weight while increasing repetitions, it is recommended to decrease the total number of sets, while keeping the weights above 80% 1RM. For instance, if performing 6 sets of 3-5 at the end of the off-season, by simply cutting back to 2-3 sets at the same rep bracket, an athlete can ensure at the very minimum, strength maintenance.

By controlling volume, the muscular and nervous systems are more apt to recover adequately, leaving the trainee fresh for future workouts, practices, and competition.

Recovery and Supercompensation

According to world renowned former Soviet strength coach Anatoly Bondarchuk, "*when discussing the nature of adaptation and its importance to performance improvement, one should always remember that training loads of differing volume and intensity evoke various change that are accompanied by specific nervous system fatigue, which temporarily reduces the body's functional abilities. It's accompanied not only by recovery (compensation) of exhausted reserves, but also by over-recovery (supercompensation), which produces the increased functional potential that lead to improved performance [1].*"

Gains can be made during the recovery period from a workout. Trainees may see gains in performance during a workout, but these are the result of adequate recovery and adaptation from previous training sessions. During and after an intense workout there is an initial breakdown of muscle proteins and depletion of energy stores, leaving the body in a state of fatigue post workout.

To bring the body back to baseline levels or beyond, hormonal adaptations, increases in protein synthesis, and nervous system recovery is required. If an athlete allows for complete recovery and structural remodeling prior to the next workout, they can achieve what is known as supercompensation. This is the goal of any training protocol. If recovery is inadequate, the athlete runs the risk of leaving the door open to the potentially negative effects of overtraining.

Some strength coaches and exercise scientists have advocated general guidelines for monitoring fatigue levels. Though not an exact science, some of these guidelines include:

- Periods of high/moderate volume followed by brief periods of low volume

- Exercise according to how your body is feeling that particular day. During the warm up, if the bar is feeling heavier than usual, it may be a day to back off on the volume or take the day off from training.

- Monitor sleep quality. Trouble staying asleep, falling asleep, or waking up can be a sign of under-recovering or overtraining.

- Monitoring resting heart rate.

- Author of Science of Sports Training, Thomas Kurz, recommends measuring grip strength first thing in the morning.

Strength scientists have even tried to quantify the stress levels of certain exercises and workloads in order to gain a better understanding of the fatigue induced by training. For instance, in a 1993 study in the Fitness and Sports Review International, strength scientist Menkhin introduced the concept of "functional stress"; the stress induced from a particular exercise load. Stepping outside of the traditional stress indexes of volume and intensity, Menkhin utilized the athlete's heart rate, duration of the work performed and something called pulse cost (the difference between the pulse rate immediately before and after exercise) to gain a better understanding of the functional stress of a given workout or work load [18].

Taking this concept a step further, expert sports scientist Dr. Mel Siff studied the relative and absolute energy expenditures of ranked and elite weightlifters. Based on the research of Vorobyev back in 1978, Siff found the most taxing exercises in terms of absolute energy expenditure to be the Clean and Jerk, with the Snatch Pull and bench press being the least [30].

Below are the findings:

Table 2: Absolute energy expenditure for a 1RM in different exercises by weightlifters of different qualification expressed in kJoules (based on vorobyev, 1978)

Exercise	Ranked Lifter	Elite Lifter	Mean of both
Snatch Pull	46.0	34.3	40.2
Bench Press	51.0	35.1	43.1
Press off racks	46.4	42.2	44.3
Clean Pull	51.0	38.9	45.0
Back Squat	47.3	46.0	46.6
Power Clean	53.1	47.3	50.2
Snatch	53.1	48.5	50.8
Front Squat	49.3	53.1	51.2
Clean and Press	54.8	49.3	52.1
Clean and Jerk	64.8	57.2	61.1

Siff M. **How strenuous is that exercise.** *Fitness and Sports Review International.* 28(5-6); Pp 192-194. 1993.

From this research, it is clear that the complexity of an exercise can also be a determinant for the levels of energy expenditure during a workout. Armed with this knowledge, coaches and athletes can design effective in-season programs for gaining or maintaining strength and size, while avoiding the pitfalls of overtraining and performance deterioration.

The end result of a balanced approach to training and recovery is positive muscular, endocrine, and neuromuscular adaptations. As can be seen, many factors play a role in affecting an athlete's fatigue levels during the competitive season. Knowledge of proper recovery methods can be the difference between a successful injury free season or sitting on the bench wondering what could have been.

Take home points:

- Cut back on volume of work rather than training loads/intensity to ensure maintenance or progression of strength. Conditioning during the season can be done on the field.
- For strength purposes, keep training loads above 80% 1RM during season.
- Monitor recovery and fatigue. We will discuss training schedules for different sports in further chapters.
- Maintain pre-habilitation exercises during season to keep injury potential minimized.
- Train efficiently, using compound movements including Olympic Lifts and variations, deadlifts, Front squats, split squats, chin ups, etc…

CHAPTER II

IN-SEASON STRENGTH

At a minimum, the goal for in-season training should be to maintain strength in order to maintain performance levels and avoid injury. For those looking to enhance their performance, progressive strength training throughout the season is required.

What good is it to be your strongest at the beginning of tryouts if you let those hard earned results fall by the wayside when the competitive season begins. Many strength coaches have advocated thinking of strength in terms of horsepower. The more horsepower you have in your motor the greater the acceleration and more powerful your movements will be. A decrease in horsepower may result in a decrease in the efficiency of athletic based movements.

Oftentimes, this drop in strength levels may be accompanied by an increase in injury potential. The musculature about a joint can become weakened with a lack of proper stimuli. This can then lead to a decrease in the quality of movement due to the over-recruitment of synergistic musculature. The result is an increased potential for strain on or about the joint leading to injury.

There are many ways to gain strength, as trainees adapt to different physical stressors in their own individual ways. For instance, a person with no previous weight training experience may gain strength with little stimuli when compared to an experienced lifter. Through neuromuscular adaptations alone they will get stronger and more efficient at recruiting muscle fibers and motor units [3,4]. Athletes with prior training experience may require a completely different approach.

As discussed in Chapter I, strength training below 80% of one's 1 repetition maximum can lead to decreases in strength [1,2]. To maintain or gain strength throughout the season, intensities above 80% are necessary. Performing high repetition bodyweight calisthenics and light weight resistance exercises may not be enough.

Strength qualities athletes need to be concerned with include speed strength, strength speed, absolute strength, and relative strength. Relative strength is of particular importance. Relative strength is the strength relative to one's bodyweight. The stronger an athlete is relative to their bodyweight, the greater the potential for power and acceleratory movements.

Studies have shown strength levels may actually drop with even 2 days per week of resistance training above 80% of an athlete's 1RM [6]. To gain or maintain strength during season, more training days may be required for some individuals. With regards to in-season strength training, certain guidelines should be adhered to:

- Adequate intensity to stimulate higher threshold muscle fibers

- Lower repetition ranges

- Higher relative volume of sets than hypertrophy based protocols

- Minimal time under tension

- Controlled eccentric contraction, while moving the concentric range as fast as possible.

- Explosive movements.

- Longer rest periods

When training for relative strength during season, exercises should be selected based upon efficiency and their ability to increase strength. For this reason, compound exercises are optimal.

In no particular order, the following is a listing of a few of the more effective compound exercises a coach or athlete should incorporate into an in-season ***strength*** training program:

(Descriptions and pictures in exercise technique section)

1. Power Cleans

2. Front Squats

3. Back Squats

4. Deadlift

5. Romanian Deadlift

6. Incline Barbell Bench Press

7. Flat Barbell Bench Press

8. Weighted Dips

9. Chin Ups

10. Pull Ups

11. Bent Over Barbell Rows

12. Standing Overhead Press

13. Push Press

14. Hamstring Curls

15. Barbell Bicep Curls

16. Close Grip Bench Press

Scheduling

Proper scheduling is an important factor for in-season strength training. Athletes should aim to avoid excessive muscle soreness and nervous system fatigue to ensure optimal game day performance. Rest and recuperation periods must be built into the weekly schedule of an in-season strength training program.

Workout scheduling begins with an analysis of the season that includes practice schedule, pre-season, off days, game days, season finale, and playoffs. Once the on-field practice and game schedule has been determined, the in-season strength training program is designed around this schedule, allowing for adequate rest to ensure optimal performance during competition. A practical method for designing any strength training program taught by Olympic Weightlifting Coaches and in Charles Poliquin's International Certification Program for strength coaches, is to start from the end goal and work backwards (5). In the case of many sports, the playoffs or finals are the goal.

Keeping these goals in mind, the aim of an in-season strength training program should be to perform at optimal levels throughout season and playoffs. During this time many opposing teams may be tired and weak, as they may have adhered to the light weight or complete abandonment of in-season training altogether.

In designing any in-season strength training program, another factor to take into account is the individual recovery ability of each athlete. Some athletes may push harder in the weight room or on the field, requiring greater or less emphasis on recovery. For that matter program options are important.

. One strategy for designing an in-season strength and conditioning program aimed at minimizing fatigue is to undulate the weekly schedule. By this, an athlete will train hard with slightly more volume one week, followed by an unloading week utilizing lesser volume. For example, a high school football team that plays games on Friday nights might design a program that entails alternating weeks of three lifting sessions with weeks of two lifting sessions. Sample Below:

Sample Schedule I: Friday Night Games

	Monday	**Tuesday**	**Wednesday**	**Thursday**	**Friday**	**Saturday**	**Sunday**
Week 1	**Lower Body Strength**	Off	**Upper Body Strength**	Off	Game	**Recovery Lift**	Off
Week 2	Off	**Total Body Strength**	Off	Off	Game	**Recovery Lift**	Off
Week 3	**Lower Body Hypertrophy**	Off	**Upper Body Hypertrophy**	Off	Game	**Recovery Lift**	Off
Week 4	Off	**Total Body Strength**	Off	Off	Game	**Recovery Lift**	Off

Scheduling lifts in a weekly undulating fashion can allow for quality lifting sessions with adequate recovery to avoid burnout and decreased game performance. A twice a week variation might look like this:

Sample Schedule II: Friday Night Games

	Monday	Tuesday	Wednesday	Thursday	Friday	Saturday	Sunday
Week 1	Total Body Hypertrophy	Off	Total Body Strength	Off	Game	Off	Off
Week 2	Recovery Lift	Off	Total Body Strength	Off	Game	Off	Off
Week 3	Total Body Hypertrophy	Off	Upper Body Strength	Off	Game	Off	Off
Week 4	Recovery Lift	Off	Total Body Strength	Off	Game	Off	Off

As critical as the scheduling of workouts is, the design of each workout is just as important. Volume control is critical to avoid burnout while maintaining strength, with low volume being the key during the competitive season.

Time efficient in-season workouts should take no longer than 35-45 minutes from the start of the first work set to the completion of the last set. This time constraint ensures optimal hormonal response while minimizing the potential for excess fatigue. Working out longer than an hour can create a negative hormonal environment that may compromise recovery ability, eventually leading to decreases in performance. To ensure optimal hormonal responses, short workouts are key during the season.

Below is a contrast between an off-season program and one that reflects in-season volume:

Off-Season Lower Body Workout

Exercise	Reps	Sets	Tempo	Rest Interval
A: Power Cleans from Mid Thigh	2-3	6	X0X0	180s
B1: Back Squats	3-5	6	3110	120s
B2: Prone Hamstring Curls	4-6	6	4011	120s
C1: Triple Jumper Step Ups	3-5	4	1010	90s
C2: Barbell Drop Lunges	3-5	4	3010	90s

In-Season variation of the same program

Exercise	Reps	Sets	Tempo	Rest Interval
A: Power Cleans from Mid Thigh	2-3	3	X0X0	180s
B1: Back Squats	3-5	3	3010	120s
B2: Prone Hamstring Curls	4-6	3	3011	120s
C1: Triple Jumper Step Ups	3-5	1	1010	90s
C2: Barbell Drop Lunges	3-5	1	2010	90s

The main difference between the two programs is the amount of total sets. The off-season workout consists of 34 total sets (a set is done on each leg for the single leg exercises), while the in-season version has 13 total sets. The rest intervals, tempo, and rep ranges are similar, allowing for similar intensities to be used for each exercise.

In summary, to maintain or gain strength during the season, intensities over 80% of an athlete's 1 repetition max are needed [1,2]. With lower intensities, athletes run the risk of decreasing strength levels over the course of a season. Keeping the horsepower at optimal levels is an effective way to ensure a safe and successful season.

Take home points:

- For strength results, train at 80% of 1RM or greater during the season.

- Compound exercises allow for greater efficiency and effectiveness of training.

- Practice and game schedule must be taken into account when developing in-season training schedule.

- Work backwards from playoffs when designing in-season strength training program.

- Allow for workout options as individual athletes may have different recovery abilities.

- Use low volume to ensure adequate recovery.

CHAPTER III

MAINTAINING WEIGHT

During the early off-season time is spent trying to correct muscular imbalances that may have occurred during the competitive season. Whether the result of decreased movement quality, overuse patterns, chronic or acute pains, or injuries, there are many reasons why these imbalances might occur. No matter the cause, finding the solution and correcting the underlying problem should be a priority.

It may not be safe for an un-trained athlete to go from their last competitive event right to heavy deep squats the following day. The risk of injury may be high and the athlete may need time to recover both his/her neuromuscular system from the rigors of the competitive season. A safe alternative might be unilateral squat variations such as split squats. Unilateral exercises can re-educate proper movement while decreasing the potential for cheating or excessive loading of the dominant side.

The same approach to correction of muscular imbalances that is applied to early off season training can also have benefit for in-season training. Pre- or rehabilitating structural imbalances can be an effective strategy in correcting deficiencies in movement. This approach may lead to enhanced performance on the playing field.

When correcting dysfunctions and repairing muscular imbalances, it may take higher repetition ranges to engrain motor patterns. In the unhealthy athlete, when a load is too heavy, proper technique, muscle recruitment, and stabilization patterns can become compromised. This can reiterate the dysfunctional pattern and increase the potential for injury over time.

Not only do hypertrophy based rep ranges provide athletes with enough resistance to increase lean muscle mass, but they also allow a light enough resistance to improve movement quality.

The following are examples of unilateral exercises that can be used for correction or prevention of muscular imbalances. These exercises fall under the weight maintenance chapter because they can be used for correction of structural imbalances rather than maximal strength or power purposes: (*see exercise technique section for description and pictures*)

1. Split Squat Variations:

2. Peterson Step Ups:

3. Box Step Ups:

4. Lunge Variations

5. Hamstring Curl Variations:

6. Single arm standing overhead dumbbell press

7. Rotator Cuff Variations

8. Bent over Dumbbell Rows

9. Dumbbell Bench Press

10. Incline Dumbbell Bench Press

11. Dumbbell Bicep Exercises

Hypertrophy

Contractile protein (myofibrillar) hypertrophy is the increase in the contractile elements involved in the generation of force and muscle tension. With heavy relative strength based weight training an increase in the density of the myofibrils (bundles of the contractile proteins actin and myosin) leads to an increase in the size of the actual muscle fiber. [5,6]

Sarcoplasmic hypertrophy is an increase in the volume of the sarcoplasm, the cytoplasmic fluid that surrounds the myofibrils and its non-contractile elements. Unlike myofibrillar hypertrophy, the density of the contractile proteins does not change, but there is an increase in muscular size due to the increased volume of the surrounding sarcoplasm and the non-contractile elements [5].

As a season begins, it is not uncommon for athletes to lose weight. Between practice hours, games, and everyday stressors, many athletes simply cannot consume enough calories to balance out the caloric expenditure. Maintaining muscle mass can be a critical element for maintaining in-season strength.

One of the major problems with hypertrophy training is the soreness associated with greater times under tension. Due to the higher repetition counts and greater time under tension, hypertrophy training can lead to delayed onset muscle soreness. For this reason, it is recommended to schedule the hypertrophy training sessions, especially lower body, with adequate time for recovery prior to the actual competition. The following are sample schedules for athletes looking to maintain weight while playing games on Saturdays.

Schedule I

	Monday	Tuesday	Wednesday	Thursday	Friday	Saturday	Sunday
Week	Upper Body	Lower Body	Off	Core/Rotators	Off	Game	Off

Schedule II

	Monday	Tuesday	Wednesday	Thursday	Friday	Saturday	Sunday
Week	Total Body	Off	Off	Total Body	Off	Game	Active Recovery

Schedule III

	Monday	Tuesday	Wednesday	Thursday	Friday	Saturday	Sunday
Week	Lower Body	Off	Upper Body	Power	Off	Game	Off

Below are a few program examples for in season weight maintenance:

Workout I: Upper Body

Exercise	Reps	Sets	Tempo	Rest Interval
A1: Incline Barbell Bench Press	6-8	3	4111	90s
A2: Neutral Grip Chin Ups	6-8	3	3011	90s
B1: V Bar Dips	8-10	3	3211	60s
B2: Seated Face Pulls	10-12	3	3012	60s
C1: Seated Dumbbell Curls	8-10	2	4020	60s
C2: Overhead Triceps Cable Ext.	8-10	2	4020	60s

Workout II: Lower Body

Exercise	Reps	Sets	Tempo	Rest Interval
A: Power Cleans from mid thigh	2-3	3	X0X0	180s
B1: Back Squats	7-9	3	4010	90s
B2: Kneeling Hamstring Curls	6-8	3	3012	90s
C1: Drop Lunges	8-10	2	3010	60s
C2: Box Step Ups	8-10	2	1010	60s

For hypertrophy purposes, the repetition counts and time under tension are greater than those seen in strength training protocols, while the rest intervals are shorter. *(More specific programs tailored toward the needs of each individual sport are covered in later chapters.)*

Caloric consumption is just as important for maintaining weight during the season. An athlete can perform hypertrophy training all they want, but if they are not eating adequate supportive calories they may be in a constant catabolic state and begin to lose muscle. A few key points with regard to in-season weight maintenance nutrition include:

- **Meeting your protein goals:** Active athletes may need a minimum of roughly 1.2-2.0 grams of protein per *KILOGRAM* of body weight.

- **Meeting your carbohydrate goals:** Athletes who are lean or carb tolerant may be able to tolerate more carbohydrates than their non-lean counterparts. For this reason an individualized approach to carbohydrate consumption may be best. If an athlete is consuming enough fat and protein and begins losing weight and muscle during the season, more carbohydrates may be necessary. If athletes begin to accumulate body fat, they may need to moderate carb intake during season. UCAN Superstarch is a great option for athletes looking to maintain muscle while minimizing the potential to gain fat during the competitive season. Their website is www.generationucan.com.

CHAPTER IV

IN-SEASON POWER

Increased power is one of the primary reasons for all the hard off-season work. This beckons the question: Is it appropriate to perform power training during the season? Rationale against power training during season may include:

- Taxing on the nervous system
- Practice may consist of power based athletic movements including sprinting, cutting, and jumping.
- Is it more appropriate to focus on strength and hypertrophy training
- Athlete may not have proper technique, therefore risking unnecessary injury

Now that we have seen some of the cons, let's look at some of the pros of in-season power training:

- Increases power and strength
- Highly efficient
- Can strengthen the nervous system if proper recovery is present
- Can train the entire body with just one lift
- Promotes muscular balance
- Teaches the body to absorb impact while increasing joint integrity for injury prevention
- Expresses powerful triple extension movement
- Promotes hip and shoulder girdle flexibility

If an athlete has worked hard in the off-season preparing the body for the rigors of the upcoming season, it may be safe to assume that resistance training has been a staple of their weekly regimen. Strength is the foundation upon which power can be built. A strong body may be more effective at maintaining stability while tapping into a greater rate of force development. Sprinting, jumping, and acceleratory movements that are done in practice and game play can be viewed as on-field methods that reflect power capabilities. But, are these movements enough to maintain or even enhance the results earned from hours of off-season training?

In athletics, explosiveness can be regarded as the ability to generate as much force as possible in as little time as possible, otherwise known as the rate of force development, or power. When we think of explosiveness, one physical action that comes to mind is the vertical jump. I have heard Division I Football recruiting coaches express that the two most important factors besides game film when deciding who to recruit are 1: How the potential recruit treats their mother and 2: How high the athlete can jump. In fact, studies have linked performance in the vertical jump to short distance sprint capability. Those athletes who had higher vertical jumps, often had better performances in the short distance acceleration sprints (3,12,13),

One of the most effective methods of increasing an athlete's vertical jump is to increase their foundation of strength and focus on increasing power. Studies have shown that athletes who performed better in the squat jump exercise also had better performances in the linear sprints (13). In an interesting study out of the Journal of Sports Medicine and Physical Fitness, researchers had subjects go through a battery of four tests, consisting of jumps, sprints, isometric strength tests, and anaerobic power testing. The researchers found correlation between performance in the depth jump and their ability to sprint 35 meters (3). In a separate study, researchers drew similar findings when testing for correlation between 5 meter sprint performance and an athlete's performance in the split squat jump (12).

Besides conventional strength training, are there any other methods of enhancing an athlete's explosive capabilities that can be used during season? A staple of many collegiate strength and conditioning programs, Olympic Weightlifting promotes explosive triple extension, similar to biomechanical movement of accelerating and jumping. The Olympic lifts consist of the Snatch and the Clean and Jerk. Modified versions of these exercises are performed from various start or catch positions.

Athletes and strength coaches have used these exercises for decades due to their efficiency, explosive characteristics and ability to develop powerful triple extension. Making gains in these lifts during season can be elusive for some athletes as these can be taxing on an already fatigued nervous system. For this reason low volume high quality of movement needs to be emphasized.

A great quality of Olympic Weightlifting is efficiency. With just one lift, an athlete is able to recruit a high number of muscle fibers. It may be the most compound of compound exercises. When done properly, the muscles of the posterior chain, (glutes, hammies, low and mid back, calf musculature) are all activated to initiate the pulling movement. Upon completion of the second pull, the catch involves a deep squat or half squat, requiring the muscles about the core, back, shoulders, quadriceps, and hips to catch the weight and then concentrically drive the weight upward in a front or overhead squat.

Will the Olympic lifts have an effect on on-field performance? Studies on strength, Olympic Weightlifting performance and their correlation to on field performance have shown that those athletes demonstrating greater abilities in the Olympic lifts and front squat also had more favorable scores in on-field biomarker tests [7,10]. Studies have also shown that the stronger the athlete, the better their performance in the Olympic Lifts [14].

In 2008 researchers looked at the short sprint and 5 yard agility performance of Australian Rules football players. The researchers found that those athletes who had better performances in the power clean and front squat also had better scores in the agility and 20m sprints [7]. When comparing Olympic Weightlifting to jump training, researchers found that Olympic Weightlifting was the training paradigm that produced a greater transfer for enhancing on field performance markers, in particular increased performance in short burst accelerations [15].

Not only have Olympic lifts been associated with dramatic increases in strength and power, but their effects on androgenic hormone production are vastly under appreciated. These total body explosive lifts have been shown to have positive effects on androgen hormones and strength gains [5]. Olympic lifts are one of the most efficient methods of optimizing ones strength, power and metabolism.

One oft-overlooked element of the Olympic lifts is their ability to create and improve flexibility. From the initial starting position which requires hamstring flexibility and low back mobility, to the catch which requires flexibility about the hips, shoulders, and back, these lifts are an excellent method of actively training flexibility.

Olympic Lifts also have the ability to injury proof the body. From the full range of motion muscle development to the increased mobility/flexibility, these lifts create strong, healthy bodies.

Olympic Weightlifting Technique

The pulling technique of the snatch and clean are very similar, both requiring triple extension, double knee bend, and a catch. The clean entails a relatively narrow grip while the snatch utilizes a wide grip. The bar is caught over the head during the snatch compared with catching the bar the clavicular area of the shoulders in the clean. A lower hip placement can be seen in the start position of the snatch due to the wider hand placement. This may also affect the point at which the bar contacts the thigh during the second pull.

General breakdown of the technique for Clean and Snatch:

Clean

Start Position

- Feet shoulder width apart with toes pointed slightly out. Feet should be flat on the ground, with pressure toward the balls of the feet.
- Back should be arched or flat with bar directly over the middle of your foot.
- Hips should be higher than the knees
- Shoulders and knees should be out over or past the bar.
- Hands are roughly shoulder width on the bar, with elbows turned out and wrists slightly flexed.
- Head should be neutral, focusing on a point straight ahead.

1st pull:

- Maintaining neutral or arched back, roughly 45 degree angle at the torso, the bar is raised by extending the knees, keeping the same torso angle relative to the ground. Try not to raise the hips first, rather maintain the same torso angle, focusing on the shoulders raising at the same time as the hips.

- The shoulders remain over the bar, with elbows turned out and wrists remaining slightly flexed.

Second Knee Bend:

- This occurs between knee and mid thigh, with a re-bending of the knees (this is the second knee bend of the double knee bend) creating a mild "unloading" effect.
- The bar is then pulled to mid-thigh.

Second Pull:

- The hips are powerfully extended
- The feet plantar flex, pushing the toes and balls of the feet into the ground.
- The shoulders are shrugged toward the ears
- Elbows are still rotated outward with wrists trying to hold flexed position.

The Catch:

- The body drops under the bar into a front squat or power position maintaining a neutral/lordotic posture
- Elbows are thrown forward with bar landing on shoulders
- Heel foot strike to ensure feet land flat on the ground.
- Eyes looking straight ahead with head neutral.

Variations:

- "Hang" refers to variations in start positions ranging from below the knee, above the knee, mid-thigh, etc..
- Power Clean refers to a catch that does not result in deep front squat, with the tops of the thighs above parallel. This exercise is more common in training and testing for sport.
- "From the blocks" refers to a start position directly off a measured box height.

Snatch

Start Position

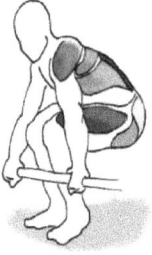

- Feet shoulder width apart with toes pointed slightly out. Feet should be flat on the ground, with pressure toward the balls of the feet.

- Back should be arched or flat with bar directly over the middle of your foot.
- Hips should be higher than the knees
- Shoulders and knees should be out over or past the bar.
- Hands are wide with hook grip, elbows turned out and wrists slightly flexed.
- Head should be neutral, focusing on a point straight ahead.

1st pull:

- Maintaining neutral or arched back, roughly 45 degree angle at the torso, the bar is raised by extending the knees, keeping the same torso angle relative to the ground. Try not to raise the hips first, rather maintain the same torso angle, focusing on the shoulders raising at the same time as the hips.
- The shoulders remain over the bar, with elbows turned out and wrists remaining slightly flexed.

Second Knee Bend:

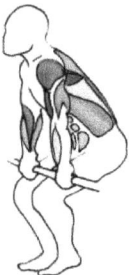

- This occurs between knee and mid-thigh, with a re-bending of the knees (this is the second knee bend of the double knee bend) creating a mild "unloading" effect.
- The bar is then pulled to mid-thigh.

Second Pull:

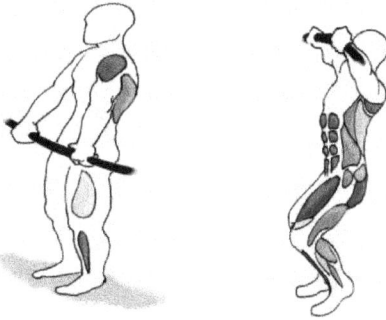

- The hips are powerfully extended
- The feet are plantar flexed pushing the toes and balls of the feet into the ground.
- The shoulders are shrugged toward the ears
- Elbows are still rotated outward with wrists trying to hold flexed position.

The Catch:

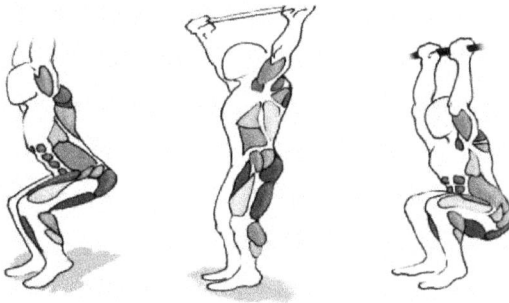

- The body drops under the bar into overhead squat
- Arms are locked straight, with the bar overhead.
- Arms are externally rotated
- Active Shoulders

- Heel foot strike to ensure feet land flat on the ground.
- Eyes looking straight ahead with head neutral.

Variations:

- "Hang" refers to variations in start positions ranging from below the knee, above the knee, mid-thigh, etc..
- Power Snatch refers to a catch that does not result in deep overhead squat, with the tops of the thighs above parallel. This exercise is more common in training and testing for sport.
- "From the blocks" refers to a start position directly off a measured box height.

Plyometric Exercises

During the days of Eastern Bloc Olympic dominance, the Soviet teams were supposedly using top secret training methods to create world and Olympic champions. Some U.S. coaches were invited to the Soviet Union to observe these secret training methods.

What they saw were athletes jumping onto and off of platforms, pushing against walls on swing like devices, throwing weights into the air from many different positions, jumping up and grabbing targets suspended from the ceiling, and many other secret training methods. Many of these movements had one thing in common: explosive movement.

Yuri Verkoshansky termed what these coaches were witnessing "shock training". Excited, these coaches went back to the U.S. and began incorporating these methods, many of which became known as "Plyometrics".

Plyometrics in the U.S. seemed to evolve from the original "shock training" to any type of jump training. Eventually anything involved with jumping seemed to fall under the plyometric umbrella. Then, the "more is better" mentality began to slowly creep in, and sub maximal Plyometrics were born. According to the late Mel Siff, for an exercise to be a true (maximal) plyometric exercise it must meet the following 5 criteria [11]:

1. **Initial Momentum Phase:** This is the initial movement of the body or body parts.

2. **Electromechanical Delay Phase:** (Eccentric Contraction) This is the time delay between motor nerve excitation and actual muscle contraction when contact is made against an immovable surface.

3. **Amortization Phase:** (Isometric Contraction) The phase in which the movement rapidly switches from eccentric to concentric muscle contraction. There is a stretch reflex that occurs in the musculotendinous unit similar to the stretching or mechanical deformation of a trampoline as you land on the surface..

4. **Rebound Phase:** (Concentric Contraction) This is the release of the energy, or the rebound force generated from the stretch reflex. As in the trampoline example, once full stretch has been reached, the elastic energy then accelerates upward in the opposite direction (release of kinetic energy).

5. **Final Momentum Phase:** (Excluding Depth Drops) Once the concentric contraction is complete the body will continue to move because of the release of the elastic energy and force generated from the concentric contraction [11]".

Plyometrics directly train the musculotendinous system of the kinetic chain. Specifically the large tendons and muscles of the body. Have you ever noticed how the highest jumping and fastest animals such as kangaroos, greyhounds, antelope, and cheetah have one thing in common? They all have very long Achilles tendons, with minimal calf muscle hypertrophy? Humans have somewhat shorter and thinner Achilles tendons with considerably larger calf musculature. Now compare human jumping capabilities to those of a kangaroo. This difference comes from multiple factors, but one is the difference in the Achilles tendon's ability to store elastic energy.

From the criteria provided by Siff, the terms maximal and sub maximal can be used to distinguish between different types of plyometric activity. Maximal Plyometrics consist of large forces being absorbed creating high levels of musculotendinous tension. These forces can then be stabilized and released in the opposite direction.

Maximal Plyometrics include depth drops and depth jumps. Sub maximal Plyometrics include low cone jumps, low box jumping, low squat jumps, ankle hops, skater hops, etc…

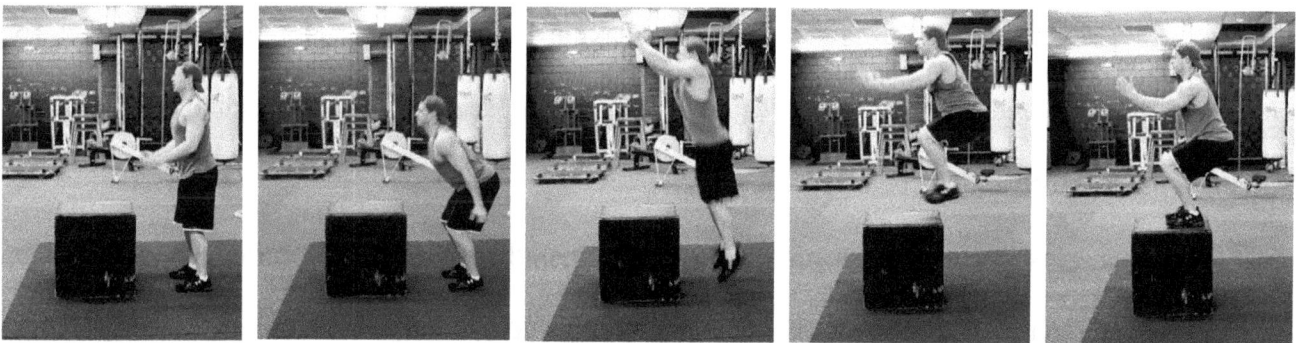

Depth Drops and Depth Jumps

Depth Drops and Depth Jumps are two of the primary forms of maximal "shock training. The ability to absorb impacts, and the ability to absorb impact and immediately generate force in the opposite direction are the foundation for these training methods.

To Perform a Depth Drop, stand on a box (the height to be determined by training experience/lower extremity strength or vertical jump height). Step forward and fall off the box. You should fall out roughly the distance equal to the height of the box. Land softly, minimizing knee bend and torso flexion, trying not to allow the weight to shift completely to the heels upon impact. Stick the landing for 3-5 seconds. Take a minimum of 1-minute rest between each jump.

A Depth Jump requires you to stand on a box (the height to be determined by training experience/lower extremity strength or actual vertical jump height) with hands behind you in the propulsive phase position of jumping. Step forward and fall off the box. You should fall out roughly the same distance as the height of the box. (If you are standing on a 24" box you should land roughly 24" away from the box). Think about jumping before you land. A good tip is to think of the ground as a hot stove as you will burn your feet if you are on the ground for too long. As soon as you land, minimize knee bend, torso flexion, and heel contact with the ground. Immediately jump up, swinging the arms upward while extending at the hips, knees, ankles, and torso.

Volume of Plyometrics is important in order to produce the desired results. When it comes to increasing the rate of force development, hundreds of repetitions of sub maximal Plyometric exercise may not elicit the same effect as $1/20^{th}$ the amount of properly executed maximal Plyometrics. If you want to jump higher and accelerate faster, performing exercises to maximize power output is a good strategy. If you want to jump low hundreds of times or accelerate at a marathon pace, performing hundreds of repetitions of sub maximal plyometrics may be a good strategy.

Ask yourself a question, would you rather run like a marathon runner or a 100m sprinter (nothing against marathon runners, this book is about increasing power output). A marathon runner is a sub maximal athlete with much less force generated per take off phase of each foot strike, while a sprinter is a maximal athlete, capable of absorbing and generating tremendous amounts of force with each phase of foot strike and takeoff. The average vertical leap of a marathon runner has been said to be roughly 12-15" whereas the average for elite 100m sprinters is roughly 34-40"+. As a team sport athlete, which would you rather have?

Hint: Using an overhead goal for plyometric training can increase adherence and enhance training result. Specific training tools like the Superupz JumpBall or a Vertec vertical jump tester are great training tools. *

Kettlebell Swing

Like most any other exercise, the mechanics and success of the movement depend heavily on the body positioning at the beginning and throughout the movement. Begin with a lordotic posture in the spine, chest out, shoulder pulled back, eyes straight ahead, and knees bent roughly 20 degrees to activate the hip extensor mechanism. Try to keep the weight over the rear of the foot. Bending at the waist rather than low back, can ensure muscle tension in the glutes and hamstrings. Hold the kettlebell with two hands, palms down. Swing the bell between the legs, just above mid shin height. At the point of full tension on the glutes and hamstrings, and the bell back behind the knees/shins, begin the upward acceleration.

The upward pull is initiated through the glutes and hamstrings, while keeping the torso in lordotic/neutral posture. Begin by swinging the weight outward and upward, raising and extending the hips, extending the knees, increasing the torso angle, and bringing the bell in an arcing movement to chin height or up above your head, while keeping the arms extended. A good tip is to contract glutes to ensure proper hip extension. At the top of the movement, stabilize the bell and allow it to swing downward in the same arcing manner. At the point of full tension in the glutes and hamstrings (bell behind the knees/shins) try to immediately change the direction again, accelerating into an upward explosive swing.

Medicine Ball Viking Throw

These should be performed outdoors on a field with lots of space or in a facility with very high ceilings. Begin the movement by positioning the body similar to the start position of the kettlebell swing. Be sure to bend at the knees and waist when positioning into the start position. This ensures the muscle tension is created in the glutes and hamstrings, rather than the low back.

Grab the med ball with two hands, palms facing each other. Swing the ball between the legs, about shin height. At the point of full tension on the glutes and hamstrings, and the ball back behind the knees/shins begin the upward acceleration. The upward pull is initiated through the glutes and hamstrings. Swing the ball outward and upward, extending the hips, extending the knees, increasing

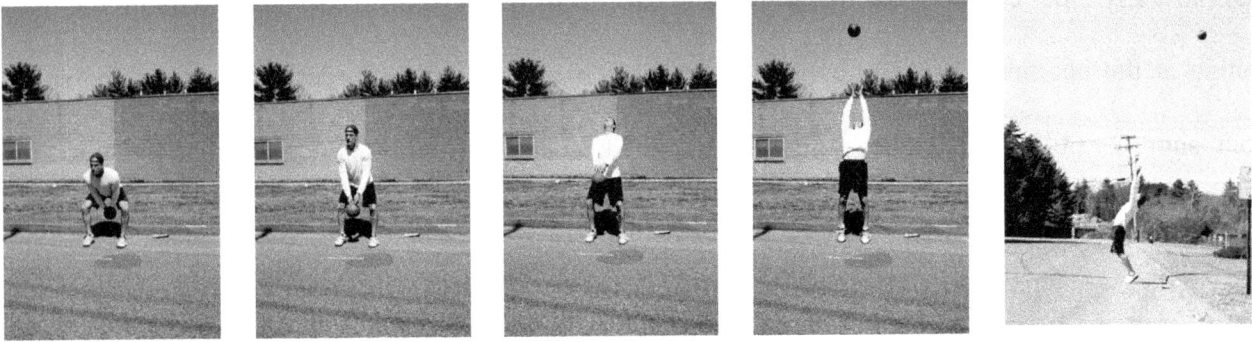

the torso angle. Swing the ball in an arcing fashion above your head, keeping the arms extended, and end on the toes. At the top of the movement, release the ball upward and backward, aiming for roughly a 45 degree trajectory. A good tip is to follow the path of the ball with your eyes to ensure optimal mechanics.

CHAPTER V

IN-SEASON FUNCTIONAL STRENGTH

Modified strongman training can be a very effective tool in building functional strength in athletes. When used properly, this type of training can increase low back strength, upright stability, grip strength, lactate tolerance, connective tissue integrity, and mental capacity.

No longer a training method typically reserved for 300+ pound strength athletes, modified versions of strongman have quietly crept into mainstream training methodology with remarkable results. Mainstream commercial health clubs have added variations of strongman training including sandbag carrying, farmer carries, sled drags, hand over hand rope pulls, and tire flipping. Elite performance training centers geared toward the highest level of athletics utilize many of the above in conjunction with cutting edge programming to create a foundation for optimal athletic performance.

Strongman training is functional training in its purest form. It has been said to bridge the gap between the weight room and on-field performance. By focusing on non-isolated, multi-segmental movements, the transfer effect to the field can be very high.

Activation of core musculature is greater in strongman exercises than many horizontal based "core" exercises as the force vector is vertical, straight down through the kinetic chain. While the abdominals do play a role in static trunk stabilization, it is the co-activation of the abdominal muscular and erector spinae musculature that creates enhanced stability in an upright position. In upright stabilization, the abdominal/oblique muscles are merely a part of a looping system; when contracted, the anterior carriage muscles create intra-abdominal pressurization that leads to spinal stability [4].

Without abdominal/oblique, hip, and spinal erector co-activation, stability is potentially unattainable. In today's sports world, heavy emphasis is placed on anterior abdominal training, while neglecting the spinal erectors. This can effectively lead to a breakdown in the body's overall stability, especially in an upright position.

By focusing their efforts on standing, load bearing, and preferably dynamic means of training, athletes can achieve a greater transfer of training effect. An excellent study by Dr. Stuart McGill and colleagues, set out to establish trunk musculature activation of Strongman training modalities. Dr. McGill and his team found tremendous supporting evidence toward the usage of upright loaded strongman exercises and transferable activation of the "core" musculature (4).

In this study, peak muscle activation of the rectus abdominis, internal and external obliques was found in all of the events, but was found to be *highest in the walking phase of the Farmer Walk, Super Yoke Walk, and the Suitcase Carry* (4). A separate study from 2007 had similar findings with regards to trunk activation and object holding/carrying. 11 male subjects had to walk between 1.9 and 3.3 mph while carrying a barbell at 3 different heights and then a bucket of potatoes at 3 different heights. The researchers found 33%, 49%, and 47% increase in erector spinae musculature in the walking barbell group versus the standing barbell group. *The walking group also had a 51% and 65% greater activation in the rectus abdominis and external oblique when compared to standing Group* (1). Of even greater significance was the abdominal activity of the group walking with the bucket of potatoes. The researchers found a *132% increase in rectus abdominis activity in the walking group compared with the standing group* (1). When walking with the bucket at knuckle or elbow height there was a two fold increase in rectus abdominis activity (1).

Conventional lifts such as squats and deadlifts have also been shown to have greater core activation than many of the now popular horizontal "core" stabilization exercise. Hamlyn et al (2007) performed a comparison study between squats, deadlifts and 30s horizontal isometric holds on trunk musculature activation. The researchers *found a statistically significant greater activation of the "core" musculature when performing 80% 1RM squats and dead lifts compared to 30s horizontal isometric holds* (2).

Along with increasing an athlete's upright stability on the field of play, strongman training also:

- Increases in lower back strength
- Increases in core strength in an upright position
- Eccentric loading and VMO strengthening during walking exercises
- Increases in ankle stability

- Increases in grip strength

- Strengthening of connective tissue

- Positive effects on bone density

- Increases in neuromuscular efficiency of synergistic muscles involved in upright stability

- Increases in functional strength of the hip flexors and extensors

- Increases in lactic and alactic capacity

- Mental toughness….

Transfer of Training

With most team sports taking place in an upright, standing, dynamic environment on a stable or immovable surface, why is it so much of mainstream "core" training takes place on squishy balance devices or in horizontal based positions? For true upright stability, weight training, combat sports, and functional strongman methods are some of the most effective methods. In **healthy athletes**, counting the dust particles on the floor while holding their body in a horizontal isometric position may not be the most time efficient, or for that matter, most effective method of increasing functional strength and upright stability. Ask yourself this question: Who would you rather try tackling on the football field, former World's strongest man Mariusz Pudzianowski or the current world record holder in plank hold?

Conventional strength exercises including squats and deadlifts at 80% of one's 1 rep max have been found to have statistically significant muscle activation of the core musculature when compared to horizontal isometric core targeted exercises [2]. Other studies have shown that *walking with a load further increased rectus abdominis activation by 132%,* when compared to standing [1]. All the more reason to include strongman protocols into your training regimen.

Recovery and Workload

Strongman training can be very taxing on the nervous system, especially when added to the cumulative fatigue of daily practices, workouts, and game preparation. Careful consideration must be taken when mapping out exercises, workload, and scheduling. Recuperation and regeneration time is paramount during the season as athletes do not want to be physically or emotionally drained heading into a competition.

If performed during any in-season protocol, recommendations for incorporating strongman include:

- Substitute strongman exercises for conventional strength exercises during lifting days. For example, tire flips could be substituted for deadlifts, hand over hand rope pulls could be substituted for rowing or chinning exercises.

- The trainee can perform one to two strongman exercises at the end of a lifting session. Sled dragging, prowler pushing, or farmer carries are good finishers.

- Strongman exercises can be used during practice. Teams may use tire flips, sled accelerations, or farmer carries during training time to create a competitive environment.

- Teams or athletes can plan an "events" day. Here the athlete(s) will incorporate multiple strongman protocols in a competition style set up. For example, an athlete may choose a tire flip, keg carry and sled drag medley. After an all-out timed set, the athlete may then rest until complete recovery. Next they may perform a hand over hand rope pull for time. Rest until full recovery. A heavy farmer carry for distance. Rest until full recovery. And lastly a keg loading sequence.

Caution should be taken in planning out events days as they are especially taxing on the adrenals and nervous system. One low volume events day per month at the max may be enough to keep the body functionally strong while minimizing adrenal stress and nervous system fatigue.

If you are concerned with under-recovering or overtraining, a simple method of testing for physical preparedness is the hand grip strength test first thing in the morning. In his book Science of Sports Training, sport scientist Thomas Kurz recommended the measurement of handgrip strength using a hydraulic dynamometer to reveal the physical readiness of an athlete (3). This information provides valuable data to the coach regarding the athlete's ability to recover from workouts.

Now that we have covered why modified strongman training is important and how to monitor if the body is recovering adequately, let's delve into some examples of modified strongman exercises and workout examples.

Strongman Exercises

- **Tire Flipping:** Often, after a difficult tire session, athletes will not only experience posterior chain soreness, but also intense forearm flexor soreness. The tire flip is an exercise in which the athlete is working the extensor muscles during the initial lifting phase, then the anterior pushing musculature to drive the tire forward and down for the next flip. Correct technique is critical in order to avoid injury. Many athletes may perform a sumo-style deadlift type movement, when in actuality safe tire flipping entails a forward motion with hands wider than feet and feet below (or somewhat behind) hips. This ensures maximal hip extensor activation with minimal risk of low back or bicep injury.

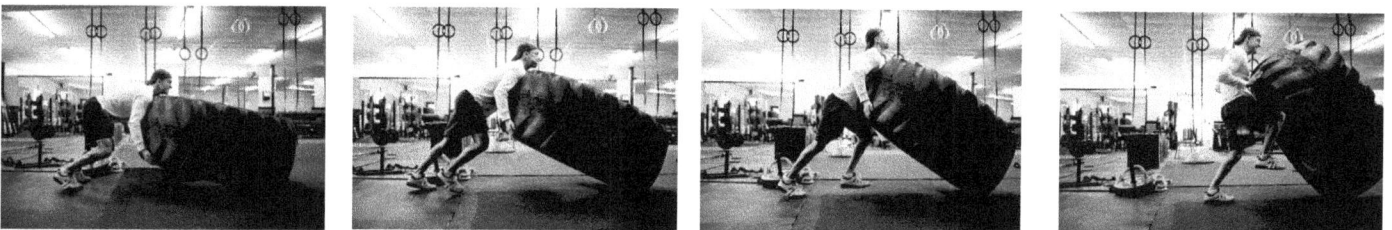

- **Super Yoke:** By focusing their time and effort on more efficient means of training, athletes can achieve a greater transfer of training effect. The methods should be upright standing, load bearing, and preferably dynamic. Recently, an excellent study by Dr. Stuart McGill and colleagues, set out to establish trunk musculature activation of Strongman training modalities. Dr. McGill and his team found tremendous supporting evidence toward the usage of upright loaded strongman exercises and transferable activation of the "core" musculature. Peak muscle activation of the rectus abdominis, internal and external obliques was found in all of the events, but was found to be *__highest in the walking phase of the Farmer Walk, Super Yoke Walk, and the Suitcase Carry__* (4).

- **Atlas Stones:** In most contact sports there is a powerful hip extensor requirement. Atlas stones are a tremendous tool (when used properly and safely) for strengthening the entire posterior chain as well as elbow flexors, core, and grip strength. The ability to lift dead weight and "pop" one's hips to elevate the stone onto or over a predetermined height can have a tremendous transfer for any contact sport.

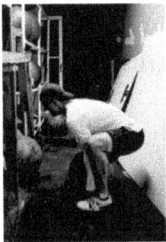

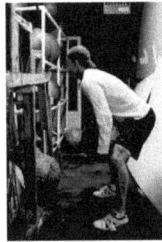

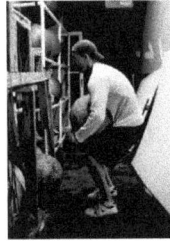

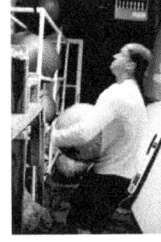

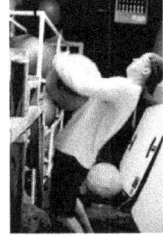

- **Axle Pulls:** Talk about a bang for your buck exercise which you can perform at any gym, with just 2 pieces of equipment: a thick bar and some plates. From entire posterior chain strengthening to enhancing grip strength, Axle Pulls are an excellent lift for any competitive athlete.

- **Farmer Carries:** Grip strength/endurance, core strength, lower extremity training, upper back and shoulder strengthening, adaptations to load bearing throughout the hips and lower extremities. The farmer carry is also great for speed development as the eccentric loading of the thigh muscles, in particular the VMO, can aid in acceleration ability.

- **Hand Over Hand Rope Pulling or Climbing:** Take a 50 foot 2-3" diameter rope and attach 300lbs to the end of it and pull hand over hand (sitting or standing with feet planted on the ground) as fast as you can. Besides the fatigue throughout the musculature in one's entire body, the lungs feel as if you have just sprinted a 400m (uphill). From grip to elbow flexors, to low back and legs, this simple but taxing exercise can build mental toughness along with all its functional strengthening benefits.

- **Sled Dragging:** This versatile tool allows for forward, backward, and lateral pulling. It can be used as a strengthening, rehabilitative, rate of force development, or metabolic conditioning tool. Whether training distance, speed, explosiveness, or strength, the benefits for the competitive athlete are numerous.

- **Keg/Sandbag Loading:** Carrying and loading asymmetrical objects has been shown to recruit up to 132% greater rectus abdominis activation than stationary standing exercises [1]. What is the significance of this for competitive athlete? Efficiency of training. While walking with an asymmetrical object, not only are you strengthening your lower body, upper and lower back, grip, and elbow flexors, but your abdominal musculature is working overtime to maintain spinal pressurization to keep the torso upright. Done for time or in medley fashion, this can be an excellent cardiovascular workout.

- **Prowler Pushes:** What contact sport competitor wouldn't want to increase their ability to generate greater amounts of force in the forward horizontal direction. The ability to explode forward/horizontally and drive your opponent backward can mean the difference between winning and losing in many contact sports. Not only can the prowler be used as a training tool for rate of force development and functional strength in the horizontal plane, but it can also be utilized as a gut wrenching metabolic conditioning tool.

- **Log Pressing:** The overhead press with the log not only develops shoulder and triceps strength, but due to its diameter, this awkward object requires tremendous activation of the abdominal, low back, and core to stabilize the body in an upright position. Be sure to roll the log up your body when racking it to the clavicles. The elbows and triceps should be pressed firmly against the lats when initiating the movement overhead. Once the log clears the forehead, to avoid excessive back strain, the head must come through the space between the arms.

- **Sledgehammer Tire Hits:** The sledgehammer tire hits are an effective tool at strengthening the musculature of the upper body and torso while working an athlete's condition. The exercise can be done with varying foot stances, one side at a time, or alternating sides.

Sample Workouts

Sample Workout I

Exercise	Reps	Sets	Rest Interval
A1: Tire Flips	2	4	0s
A2: Backward Sled Drag	20 yds	4	0s
A3: Tire Flips	2	4	0s
A4: Backward Sled Drag	20yds	4	180s
B1: Overhead Log Press	4-6	3	30s
B2: Prowler Push	20yds	3	90s

Sample Workout II

Exercise	Reps	Sets	Rest Interval
A: Axle Lifts	3-5	3	180s
B1: Farmer Carry	20yds	3	30s
B2: Overhead Log Press	6-8	3	120s
C1: Prowler Push	30yds	2	10s
C2: Backward Sled Drag	30yds	2	90s

Sample Upper Body Workout (In Season strength training workout with strongman protocols)

Exercise	Reps	Sets	Rest Interval
A1: Fat Grip Barbell Bench Press	3-5	4	120s
A2: Fat Grip Chin Ups	3-5	4	120s
B1: Dips	4-6	2	90s
B2: Bent Over Barbell Rows	4-6	2	90s
C1: Tire Battle	10	2	30s
C2: Hand over Hand Rope Pull	20yds	2	60s

Sample Lower Body Workout (In Season strength training workout with strongman protocols)

Exercise	Reps	Sets	Rest Interval
A1: Back Squats	3-5	4	120s
A2: Kneeling Hamstring Curls	3-5	4	120s
B1: Dumbbell Split Squats	4-6	2	90s
B2: Box Step Ups	4-6	2	90s
C1: Farmer Carry	20yds	2	30s
C2: Backward Sled Drag	30yds	2	60s

CHAPTER VI

IN-SEASON NUTRITION

What should I eat throughout the day of a competition? What is the best food to eat after a game? How can I maintain weight? What foods should I eat to lose weight? These are all common questions many athletes have with regards to their in-season nutrition.

The simplest way start any discussion on nutrition is to break down the three macronutrients used by the body:

- Protein

- Fats

- Carbohydrates

Protein

Protein is discussed first because in Greek terminology, the word "proteus" means first. In other words not only is protein discussed first, but trainees may want to make it their first nutritional priority. Proteins are made up of amino acids that provide the building blocks for tissue, cellular repair and health, nutrient transportation, energy, oxygen carrying capacity, hormone production, neurotransmitter production, digestion, and much more. Examples of protein include:

- Steak

- Chicken

- Fish

- Eggs

- Cheese

Essential Amino Acids

There are 8 essential amino acids your body requires for basic physiological functioning. A deficiency in any of these may lead to negative health consequences including weakened immune function, thyroid dysfunction, chronic fatigue, mental disorders, Candida, and more. Essential amino acids are those the body cannot manufacture, therefore they are required in our diets.

8 Essential Amino Acids:

Isoleucine

Leucine

Lysine

Methionine

Phenylalanine

Threonine

Tryptophan

Valine

Non-Essential Amino Acids

There are 14 non-essential amino acids that your body can manufacture itself. These are responsible for everything from brain and immune function to detoxification and digestion.

14 Non-Essential Amino Acids

Alanine

Arginine

Asparagine

Aspartic Acid

Cysteine

Glutamic Acid

Glutamine

Glycine

Histidine

Proline

Serine

Tyrosine

Branched Chain Amino Acids

The BCAAs include Valine, Leucine, and Isoleucine. These have been found in studies to have beneficial effects on protein synthesis post physical exercise [1,2]. BCAAs may also aid in minimizing muscle protein breakdown and as well as optimizing hormonal response during exercise.

Not all protein sources are the same

There is a large debate over the necessity of organic and grass fed proteins versus non-organic and often times processed proteins. The nutritional values of each can be on opposite ends of the spectrum with regards to impact on our health.

Benefits of Organic Grass Fed Proteins:
- No hormones or antibiotics used to treat the animals, thus limiting the amount of these chemicals passed to the consumer through consumption.

- Higher levels of Conjugated Lineolic Acid.

- Higher levels of Omega 3 and 6 Fatty acids

- Less chance of E-Coli contamination

- Often times, better and cleaner taste

Best sources of protein include:
- Grass Fed Beef

- Bison

- Turkey

- Free Range organic Eggs

- Free Range Organic Chicken

- Lamb

- Coldwater fish including Herring, Sardines and

- Wild caught Salmon

Post Workout Protein Shake

Whey, Casein, Rice, and Egg protein are all quality powder protein sources. Later in this chapter there is a section on Post Workout Shakes.

Fats

Does fat actually make us fat? A simple test for this is to go two weeks without eating carbohydrates and then two weeks without eating fats and test for the fat loss results.

Is the cholesterol in our diets the same as the cholesterol in our arteries? Roughly 15% of the cholesterol in our blood comes from our food sources while the remainder is produced by the body. Serum triglycerides, or fats found in the blood, are another risk factor we need to be concerned with. These can be directly manipulated by our diets. Many functional medicine experts express the quickest way to decrease serum triglycerides (blood fats) is to go on a low carb higher fat diet.

Saturated fats can have many benefits on including:

- Hormone production

- Cell membrane health

- Clean burning sustainable fuel source

- Antioxidant properties

- Bone health

- Fat Soluble vitamin transport

- And more

Butter Vs Margarine: Science vs. Marketing

The late functional nutrition expert, Dr. Robert Crayhon, once performed a study in which he put a stick of margarine outside his window sill for a period of time. The objective was to see if any animal or bug would eat it. After a few days, not a single creature touched it. Even mold or maggot dared not go near it as even these did not view it as food.

Deciding to take this test one step further, we put three sticks of margarine in three different locations: one in a dumpster, one right next to an ant colony, and one in the woods near some animal tracks. Next to each of these was a stick of organic butter. Within a matter of days, the butter was completely gone, while the margarine was untouched.

From these experiments one beckons to ask the question: if animals and bugs won't even touch margarine, then why is it OK for us to eat it?

The Beauty of Butter

Is butter as bad as many would have us think? It depends on who you listen to. Yes butter is a source of fat, but is the fat in butter all that bad? For example, butter is high in all fat soluble vitamins, contains Conjugated Linoleic and Butyric acid, and helps in the absorption of vitamin D.

Fats to Stay Away From

Trans or Hydrogenated Fats: These fats are associated with increased inflammation and risk of heart attack as they are high in omega 6 fatty acids.

Carbohydrates

Carbohydrates are broken down into blood sugar, and can be used for both short term and moderate term energy. The three types of carbohydrates include:

- Monosaccharide

- Disaccharides

- Polysaccharides

Do We Need Carbohydrates to Function

Did you know there is no such thing as an essential carbohydrate? We have essential amino acids. We have essential fatty acids. We have yet to find an essential carbohydrate. Are carbohydrates completely necessary for energy and human functioning? Understanding that the brain and heart are not glucose dependent organs, the answer becomes grayed. When carbohydrates are not present in the diet, the body begins to run off of ketones as it breaks down fatty acids for fuel.

Take for example Eskimos. Many live off of fat and protein solely. The ketones provide the brain with up to 70% of its fuel after only a few days on a low carb ketogenic diet. The heart on the other hand is very efficient at running off of fatty acids for fuel.

High glycemic carbohydrates on the other hand can spike blood sugar levels, which in turn requires more insulin to shuttle the glucose into the cells. The receptors on the cells eventually become less sensitive to the insulin, presenting a state of insulin resistance or type II diabetes.

Elevated levels of blood sugar from high glycemic carbohydrates will provide the trainee or athlete with a short-term energy boost, but once the acute energy spike drops off, there is a crash in energy levels.

Charles Poliquin expresses that consuming high glycemic carbohydrates prior to a workout can lead to an increase in serotonin production. Serotonin is the neurotransmitter associated with a calm and relaxed state. Calm and relaxed may not be the best mental state when engaging in a hard workout session. Instead, focused and driven may be more appropriate.

Post workout carbohydrates

In theory, carbohydrates immediately post workout can be an effective strategy in bringing the body back to an anabolic state and speeding up muscle protein remodeling after an intense weight training workout. Carbs can replenish glycogen supply, potentially enhancing recovery and muscle growth. Some research though, has shown carbohydrates may not be necessary post workout, as the protein consumed immediately post workout may be enough to enhance protein synthesis.

Pre Workout Nutrition Ideas

As previously mentioned, in his teachings, world renowned strength coach Charles Poliquin expresses that foods that enhance drive and ability to concentrate should be a priority pre-workout. The neurotransmitters associated with these are dopamine and acetylcholine. As we saw earlier, carbohydrates may not be the best option for this neurotransmitter response, as they increase serotonin production. Instead, foods that enhance dopamine and acetylcholine production include:

- Coldwater fish

- Cottage Cheese

- Avocado

- Nuts (not peanuts as these are legumes)

- Steak cooked in butter

- Salba

- Total fat Greek yogurt

Tip: Try a grass fed steak cooked in organic butter 2-3 hours prior to strength testing.

Pre- workout foods that may not be the best option with regards to optimal neurotransmitter response as well as water being pulled into the digestive tract include:

- Bagel

- Oatmeal

- Cereal

- Low fat yogurt

- Chips, popcorn, and crackers

- Rice cakes

UCAN

This SuperStarch represents the next level of sustainable fuel sources. With little effect on insulin, UCAN actually spares glycogen depletion while promoting utilization of fat stores as energy. Imagine drinking a shake before a game that provides sustainable fuel, burns fat, has no effect on insulin, while promoting blood sugar stability. UCAN is currently being used by many athletes from the highest levels of professional sports. For more on this tremendous product, check out www.generationucan.com.

Post Workout Nutrition Ideas

One of the most efficient and effective strategies for delivering a high glycemic, high antioxidant, high protein meal, is to consume a post workout, liquid protein shake. Liquid meals have been shown to be assimilated by the body much faster than a solid meal. Fruits and fruit juices including blueberries, prunes, blackberries, raspberries, cherries, and pomegranates provide antioxidants to protect the body from free radicals produced during the workout.

Sample post workout nutrition:

- 20-30 grams quality whey protein mixed in water.

- Glutamine

- A Greens powder mix is an effective strategy to re-alkalize the body after a workout.

- A handful of high antioxidant fruits including blueberries, blackberries, cherries, or prunes.

Whether weekend warriors, off-season athletes, or in season competition, optimal nutrition is an integral part of athletic preparation. Without proper nutrition, on-field performance can be hindered and results can stagnate. In order to move forward, nutrition cannot be left behind.

Top 10 Foods for In-Season Training

1. Grass Fed Beef
2. Organic Duck Eggs
3. Blueberries
4. Wild Caught Salmon
5. Avocado
6. Nuts
7. Steel Cut Oatmeal
8. Quinoa
9. Cherries
10. Organic Butter

In-Season Snack Ideas

Weight Maintenance

Anabolic Brownies

Gluten Free Brownie Mix

3 Scoops Chocolate Casein Protein Powder

2 pouches of UCAN

4 free range organic eggs

1 stick of organic butter

Greek Yogurt Treat

Total Fat Greek Yogurt

Chocolate Whey or Casein Protein Powder

Cinnamon

Chia Seeds

Blueberries

Cherries

Gluten Free Organic French Toast

Gluten Free Cinnamon Raisin Bread

Organic Free Range Eggs

Cinnamon

Vanilla Extract

Pancakes

Gluten Free Pancake Mix

Vanilla Whey Protein Powder

Organic Butter

Organic Apple Slices

Organic Banana

Rice Cakes

Organic Brown Rice Cakes

Almond Butter

Organic Raspberry Jam

Homemade Bison Jerky

Low Sodium Bison Jerky

Pre-Workout Snacks

UCAN

1-2 packets UCAN

Pre-workout Healthy Fat and Fiber Snack

Organic Apple

Almond Butter

Strong for Workout Snack

Organic Grass-Fed Beef cooked in organic butter

Avocado

Cognition Snack

Sardines

Coconut Oil

Mixed nuts consisting of Macadamia Nuts, walnuts, and Brazil Nuts

CHAPTER VII

IN-SEASON INJURY

MANAGEMENT

Throughout any given sports season the potential for injury exists. Whether due to acute trauma or chronic overuse, injuries can hinder athletic movements, potentially altering performance and in some cases, end a season. As the old saying states, *"an ounce of prevention is worth a pound of cure"*. This statement holds particularly true in the world of competitive sports.

When an injury does occur, athletes will typically see their trainer, doctor and depending on severity, a specialist. Anti-inflammatory methods, physical therapy, rest, or surgery may be recommended. Besides these options, are there any other strategies to manage injuries during the competitive season?

Anti-Inflammatory Diet

Approaching inflammation from the inside out can be an effective strategy in treating chronic pains. Whether due to food sensitivities, excessive inflammatory fatty acids, chemical toxicity, acidosis, or lack of anti-inflammatory nutrients, a broad spectrum of symptoms can result from excessive inflammation.

Foods known for their anti-inflammatory properties include:

Blueberries	Avocado	Kale	Wild Caught Salmon Turmeric
Cherries	Sardines	Bok Choy	Grass Fed Beef
Raspberries	Macadamia Nuts	Spinach	Coconut Oil
Papaya	Walnuts	Green Beans	Extra Virgin Olive Oil
Pineapple	Brazil Nuts	Broccoli	Cinnamon

Foods to avoid include:

Processed foods	Cereals	Fried Food	Candy Food Coloring Agents
Bagels	Dairy	Hard Cheeses	Polyunsaturated Vegetable Oils
Margarine	Fast Food	Potato Chips	Improperly Fermented Soy Products

Hydration and Electrolytes

During intense exercise, electrolytes may become depleted through sweat. Dehydrated tissue can become weak, rigid, and susceptible to injury. Without proper hydration, blood flow and repair capabilities can be compromised. Restoring these electrolytes is critical for restoring tissue hydration.

Active Release Technique

The brainchild of soft tissue expert Dr. Michael Leahy, ART is a soft tissue technique that utilizes a combination of deep tissue massage and passive movement. Adhesions or scar tissue can build up inside fascial and muscle tissue leading to impairments in movement. These adhesions can be painful, oftentimes leading to avoidance of the movement or postures that trigger the pain. Compensations may result, leading to even greater potential for injury about the inflamed or other areas. For more information on Active Release Technique, check out www.activerelease.com

Self Myofascial Release

SMFR is another method of breaking up scar tissue and restoring fascial tissue back to normal length. SMFR utilizes a BioFoam roller to massage and potentially break up adhesions in the soft tissue. It can be used pre-workout, during workout, or post workout to aid in not only restoring soft tissue length, but also enhancing circulation and recovery ability while decreasing inflammation. Common techniques in include SMFR of the IT band, piriformis muscles, hamstrings, quadriceps, calves, adductors, mid back, and latissimus musculature. For low back pain, according to neuromuscular therapist Katie Adams, a Kong dog chew ball or lacrosse ball can be effective tools to palpate deeper muscles the foam roller cannot quite reach.

Fascial Stretch Therapy

Ann and Chris Frederick's trademarked Fascial Stretch Therapy focuses on restoring, enhancing, or optimizing connective tissue length through a combination of nervous system relaxation and assisted or non-assisted full range of motion stretching techniques. When utilized properly, Fascial Stretch Therapy can restore joint range of motion, allowing for enhancement of movement quality and efficiency. Fascial stretching can be done at the end of a workout as it can also aid in recovery due to the enhanced blood flow to the active muscles. For more on Fascial Stretch Therapy, it is highly recommended to check out Ann and Chris Frederick's Stretch To Win at www.stretchtowin.com

Microcurrent Therapy

Microcurrent therapy is a low level electrical current therapy aimed at increasing circulation and decreasing inflammation in soft tissue. Of the many benefits of Microcurrent therapy, enhancing ATP production may be one of the most important. By stimulating ATP production, Microcurrent therapy can aid in healing damaged cells. This can lead to alleviation of both chronic and acute injuries and pain.

Proteolytic Enzymes

Proteolytic enzymes, otherwise known as proteases, are enzymes that break down proteins, attacking the bonds that hold amino acids together. Some examples of these include bromelain (from pineapple), papain (from papaya), trypsin and chymotrypsin (also from pineapple), and the silk worm enzyme, otherwise known as Serratia Peptidase.

In 2004, researchers put together an excellent study on the effect proteolytic enzymes had on acute inflammation caused by running. In this double-blind, placebo controlled study the subjects were given a seven enzyme mixture 4 times per day between 24 and 96 hours after their downhill running bout, or a placebo. The enzyme group "demonstrated superior recovery of contractile function and diminished effect of DOMS [10]" compared with the group receiving the placebo. The researchers concluded that the proteolytic enzymes may enhance the healing process allowing for increased restoration of muscle function after exercise [10].

A second study, this one done in 2007, set out to test the effectiveness of proteolytic enzymes on muscle soreness resulting from eccentric loading. In this double-blind, placebo controlled study, the researchers found a much more rapid recovery from the workout as well as a decreased loss of strength immediately after the workout[4]. Not only do proteolytic enzymes aid in fighting inflammation, but they may also prevent short term post workout strength losses.

Topical Performance and Recovery Creams

When soft tissue is damaged, delivery of oxygen and nutrients to the cells can be interrupted and ATP production can be compromised. These factors can lead to a decrease in tissue healing. Ignite and Xccelerate by Zanagen Corporation are two topical creams that aid in localized tissue healing.

The Ignite is a topical pre workout vasodilator that increases microcirculatory blood flow. This enhanced blood flow to soft tissue increases the potential for valuable nutrients and oxygen to reach the desired areas. Once the circulation has been enhanced to the damaged area, the Xccelerate contains ingredients aimed at reducing inflammation, pain, and scar tissue to the damaged tissue. The Xccelerate can be used after workout, practice, or game to reduce muscle soreness and soft tissue damage.

Grip Strength

Did you know that the strength of one's grip has been associated with overall health? Often overlooked or taken for granted, the strength of one's grip can be an important factor in injury prevention and overall strength development. Grip strength can also play a key role in many sports. The football player trying to rip down an opponent, the basketball player protecting the ball, the baseball pitcher controlling their pitches, and the hockey player taking a wrist shot. They all have a need for grip strength.

The grip can often be a limiting factor in many elements of training and sport. The athlete with a weak grip may struggle during deadlifts, cleans, and chin ups. That same athlete may struggle on the field with movements and actions requiring grip strength.

Did you know that the health of one's rotator cuff has been associated with the strength of one's grip? An athlete with a weak rotator cuff may be susceptible to injury, particularly in the pressing movements. A 2005 study found a significant correlation between the muscle strength of the external rotators on the injured side and the strength of one's grip on that same side (13). In a separate study, this one from the Department of Orthopedic surgery at the Baylor College, the researchers found rotator cuff weakness on the side in which the hand was injured (5).

Omega Wave Technology

Used by college strength and conditioning programs as well as some of the world's top futbol clubs, OmegaWave allows athletes to learn if they are recovering from training loads and adapting to the rigors of the competitive season. By utilizing physiological parameters including Heart Rate Variability, Differential ECG, Omega potential, neuromuscular assessments, and work capacity testing, OmegaWave technology let's an athlete know if they are under-recovering, overtraining or ready to take the field. For more on this cutting edge technology, check out www.omegawave.com.

Hyperbaric Oxygen Therapy

Blood flow can be restricted due to inflammation. This can create difficulty for oxygen and other healing factors to reach injured sites due to the constriction of blood vessels. Hyperbaric chambers counteract this by saturating the blood and hemoglobin with oxygen. Once oxygen and red blood cells are able to reach the injured site, immune function and injury healing capacity can be enhanced.

Ayurvedic Medicine

A great remedy for inflammation is Turmeric Rhizome Extract. Particularly a compound known as curcumin, which is the primary ingredient in many Ayurvedic medicinal applications.   Acting as a potent anti-oxidant, curcumin has been found to be effective in the treatment of various illnesses including multiple forms of cancer, arthritis, Alzheimer's, and even bacterial infections such as Staph. An abundance of scientific research has shown curcumin to be effective in the treatment of chronic inflammation and the diseases associated with this inflammation.

For example, a 2009 review on both clinical and preclinical research of the anti-inflammatory properties of curcumin provided valuable insight into the actions as well as effects of this "Indian Solid Gold". Three types of curcuminoids (diferuloylmethane, demethoxycurcumin, and bisdemethoxycurcumin) were discussed by the researcher. Their benefits as antioxidants as well as antimicrobials could have positive effects on sicknesses ranging from cancer to inflammation[7]. A separate review from 2009 expressed similar findings [1].

Far Infrared Sauna Therapy

Far Infrared Sauna Therapy offers tremendous healing potential for the In-Season Athlete. By passing through the skin, far infrared treatment enhances capillary vasodilation, which in turn increases blood flow, allowing for oxygen and nutrients to reach the damaged areas. This increases soft tissue repair and recovery, while reducing the potential for infection due to the associated increase of white cell production. Far Infrared Sauna Therapy is also a very effective method of detoxification.

Contrast Shower

Regular shower hot, 60 seconds freezing cold, 60 seconds hot, and 60 seconds freezing cold. This method of showering after a practice or workout can enhance circulation, aiding the recovery process.

Active Recovery

Active recovery enhances blood flow to the working muscles, enhancing the ability to shuttle waste products out, while driving nutrients into the cells and tissue. Methods of active recovery include:

- Walking

- Yoga

- Light weight training or calisthenics

- Stationary Bike or Elliptical

- Forward Sled Dragging

CHAPTER VIII

IN-SEASON GAME DAY TIPS

Post Activation Potentiation

In the 1988 Olympics, the 100m dash came down to two heavily favored sprinters, Carl Lewis and Ben Johnson. The story ends with Johnson winning the race in world record time, but then being disqualified as he tested positive for steroids. His sprint coach, Charlie Francis, was considered to be at the forefront of maximizing human performance, in particular Olympic caliber sprinters. One of the overshadowed methods he used with great benefit was post-activation potentiation.

Post activation potentiation (PAP) is a phenomenon in which a trainee is capable of potentiating their nervous system to achieve a higher level of activation, leading to an enhanced motor unit and muscle fiber recruitment during the ensuing event.

Rumors abound about Ben Johnson squatting 600lbs for 3 reps 10 minutes prior to running a 100 meter race. In theory, the 600lb squat potentiated his nervous system, allowing high threshold muscle fibers and motor units to become active. Once active, these high threshold fibers would then be primed, allowing him to maximally contract the active musculature to rapidly accelerate down the track.

The basic theory is to acutely enhance nervous system and muscular force output. This is done by performing a heavy, high threshold muscle fiber recruitment exercise, immediately followed by an explosive movement that requires similar musculature .

A 2010 study out of the Journal of Strength and Conditioning Research studied the effects three different conditioning stimuli (3 rep max half squat, plyo, and inactivity) had on jumping ability. What they found was that after a five minute rest period, the subjects whom performed the 3 rep max half squats saw more favorable results in the countermovement jump height than plyometric exercises or rest [1].

In a separate study out of the Neuromuscular Laboratory at Appalachian State University, researchers compared the effects stimulatory effects heavy squats, loaded countermovement jumps, or rest had on 10, 30, and 40m sprint performance in college football players. After performing the stimulatory exercise followed by four minutes of rest, the subjects who performed the heavy squats first realized the best performances in the 10, 30, and 40m sprints, especially in those subjects whom were characterized as weaker per pound of body weight (5).

Example of PAP include:

- 3 rep max back squat → rest 30-45s→all out 20m sprint

- 2 rep max deadlift→rest 30-45s→vertical jump

- 2 rep power clean from hang above the knee→rest 3045s→10yd prowler sprint

- 2 rep max bench press→rest 30-45s→3 rep chest pass med ball throw for distance.

In Season Programming

Pre-Competition Nervous System Warm-up Workout

2-24 hrs prior to competition

Exercise	Rep Range	Sets	Tempo	Rest Interval
A: 5 Min warm up on bike				
B1: SMFR	15-30s per			
B2: Dynamic stretching swings	10 per			
C1: 70-80% 1Rm Power Clean from mid thigh 2 reps		2	X0X0	60s
C2: 12-24" Hurdle Hops	4	2		120s
D: Resisted Sled Sprint	15 yds	2		120s

Hamstring Circulation

This great tip was introduced to me by World Renowned Olympic Weightlifting Coach Istvan Javorek. Along with shortening the hip flexors, sitting for long periods of time can cut off circulation to the hamstring musculature. With this decreased blood flow comes a decrease in the oxygen carrying capacity of the muscles, and therefore the energy production to these muscles while they are working. Coach Javorek used to have his athletes stay off their hamstrings while sitting to minimize compression when traveling to a competition (3). For more information on Coach Javorek and his excellent book Complex Training, check out his website www.istvanjavorek.com.

Pre-Activity Nutrition

This tip comes from Coach Charles Poliquin's teachings on pre workout nutrition and the effects food has on our neurotransmitter production. The effect a food has on neurotransmitter production is key before a competition. Enhancing the drive and focus neurotransmitters is critical. For that reason it is important to eat foods that enhance dopamine and acetylcholine production while minimizing those that enhance serotonin production. Quality fats and protein enhance dopamine and acetylcholine while carbohydrates enhance serotonin.

Regarding energy for activity, fat is a much more efficient and clean burning fuel source than carbohydrates. On average, the body stores on average 40-50 times more energy as fat than it does as glycogen (7). For more on Coach Poliquin's teachings check out his website at www.charlespoliquin.com

UCAN

The UCAN SuperStarch is a waxy maize product that is processed using a proprietary heat-moisture method. This method of processing creates a slow absorbing carbohydrate source with very minimal effect on insulin oar blood sugar. Originally created for the treatment of a rare genetic disorder called glycogen storage disease, the SuperStarch allowed for more sustainable blood glucose levels and energy. Another benefit of UCAN is that it can actually enhance free fatty acid utilization during intense workouts. For more on UCAN or to order the product, check out www.generationucan.com

Pre-Activity Supplementation

Alpha GPC

Used in the treatment of post-concussion syndrome, stroke, and Alzheimer's Disease, Alpha GPC has also been used for its acetylcholine boosting effects to enhance workout drive and concentration. Alpha GPC has also been shown in research to enhance growth hormone production. Quite possibly the best Alphas GPC on the market is the Poliquin brand and can be found at www.charlespoliquin.com

Ginkgo Biloba

Known for its effects on brain and cognition, Ginkgo Biloba can also be used to enhance circulation during workouts. Ginkgo's antioxidant capacity and positive effects on blood platelets comes from compounds known as flavone glycosides. Ginkgo also contains ginkgolides and bilobalides, organic compounds known as terpenes that are known to enhance circulation to the brain.

Huperzine A

Huperzine A is another brain boosting supplement that has been used in the treatment of Alzheimer's Disease. Huperzine works by inhibiting the enzyme responsible for the breakdown of the neurotransmitter acetylcholine. This allows for a rise in the levels of the acetylcholine in the brain, which can lead to enhanced memory, focus, and concentration.

L-Tyrosine

Derived from the amino acid phenylalanine, Tyrosine (from the Greek word "tyros" for cheese as it is found in casein protein) is responsible for the synthesis of the catecholamines, the neurotransmitter dopamine, and hormones including thyroid and adrenal hormones.

Beta Alanine + Creatine

Beta Alanine is an amino acid that enhances lactic acid buffering capacity by enhancing the body's levels of Carnosine. Creatine enhances ATP energy production through increases in Creatine Phosphate levels. When taken together, an athlete can work for longer durations at higher intensities, with less fatigue.

Enhancing Muscular Activation

There are many different methods of potentially restoring muscle activity. The basic idea behind many of these techniques is to enhance the communication between the nervous system and the working muscles. Through decreasing adhesions in the soft tissue to enhancing mechanical receptor responsiveness, muscles that have had decreased activity for years may begin to awaken with these techniques. Examples of what an athlete can expect from utilizing techniques to enhance muscular activation:

- Stimulation of the Golgi tendon organ or stretch reflex to enhance the neuromuscular response

- Increasing range of motion to allow for better communication between the nervous system and active muscles

- Restoring tissue length and health to decrease blockages in the afferent and efferent signals

- Decreasing inhibition of antagonistic muscles

Optimizing Movement Quality

Introduced to me by world-renowned low back expert, Dr. Stu McGill, the concept of movement quality is an often overlooked but highly important factor in athletic preparation. Movement quality is a combination of muscular balance between antagonistic and synergistic muscle groups, optimal activation/deactivation patterns and timing of those muscle groups, efficient neuromuscular and myofascial communications, and optimal joint angles. The combination of these can lead to movements that are both fluid and efficient, while decreasing the potential for injury and increasing the potential for strength, speed, and power.

Through a combination of fascial release and stretch techniques, applied kinesiology, chiropractic, soft tissue work, oral and topical anti-inflammation products, isometric training, neuromuscular re-education, stim, postural correction exercises, and dynamic movements, athletes are able to re-educate the quality of movement they once had prior to chronic overuse and acute injuries.

Proper Warm Up

Over the past years there have been many debates on how athletes should warm up and stretch prior to activity. The original schools of thought revolved around light jogging followed by static stretching. The rationale behind this was that a stretched muscle has less chance of being injured and is therefore ready for activity. Through the increased range of motion acquired from static stretching, it was believed that an athlete could then improve performance on the field.

In reality, these athletes were actually decreasing their performance. In a 2004 study on World Class Rugby Players, researchers found a reduction in the force a muscle could generate when statically stretched prior to a twenty meter sprint. The researchers believed this was due to decreased muscle-tendon compliance and neural inhibition (2). *Below is a chart from their study with the results of the subjects 20m sprint times after different stretch modalities.*

Stretching Modality	20m Pre-Stretch Time (s)	20m Post-Stretch Time (s)
Passive Static Stretch	**3.23s**(+/- 0.17)	**3.27s**(+/- 0.17)
Active Dynamic Stretch	3.24s(+/-0.2)	3.18s(+/-0.18)
Active Static Stretch	**3.24s**(+/-0.18)	**3.29s**(+/-0.2)
Static Dynamic Stretch	3.25s(+/-0.22)	3.22s(+/-0.21)

As can be seen in the above chart, the static stretching protocols actually led to decreased times in the 20m sprint. The passive static stretch led to a loss of .04s on average while the active static stretch lost .05s on average.

A 2006 study out of the Journal of Strength and Conditioning Research tested the vertical jump, flying 20m sprint, agility, and stationary 10m sprint of professional soccer players after static, dynamic, and no stretching (4). *The results are below:*

Type of Stretching	Vertical Jump (cm)	Stationary 10m sprint (s)	Flying 20m sprint (s)	Agility (s)
Static	39.4	1.85	2.37	5.22
Dynamic	40.4	1.83	2.37	5.14
None	40.6	1.87	2.41	5.20

Interestingly, the vertical jump was best without any stretching at all prior to execution. 10m sprint and agility were slower, with the agility being significantly slower after static stretching. To account for the dramatic differences in the vertical jump, 10m sprint, and agility tests, a decrease in power may have been observed (4). According to a research article out of the National Strength and Conditioning Journal, the authors expressed that static stretching could lead to decreases in strength and power production by roughly 5-30% (8).

Dynamic stretching has become an important element of pre-activity warm-ups. If tight, muscles that act as antagonists to prime movers in sporting movement may need to be stretched statically prior to activity. For example, if the hip flexors are tight, they may lead to an inhibition of their antagonistic muscles, the hip extensors. If the hip extensors are not firing properly, this can decrease an athlete's ability to accelerate, jump, sprint, or any other sporting movement that requires great degrees of hip extension power.

THE HIP FLEXORS: Illiacus, Psoas Major, and Psoas Minor (and the rectus femoris).

- Produce hip flexion and external rotation
- Functions: Eccentrically decelerate femoral rotation at heel strike
- Eccentrically decelerate hip extension
- Assist in stabilizing the lumbar spine during functional movements

Why should an athlete statically stretch the hip flexors before activity???

Hip extension plays a major role in the propulsive force upward during jumping, or forward during sprinting and accelerating. If an athlete wants to run faster, accelerate better, or jump higher, they will need maximal activation of their hip extensors, in particular the hamstrings and gluteus maximus muscles. **If the hip flexors are tight, they can inhibit the glutes from firing maximally. This is a phenomenon known as Reciprocal Inhibition.**

FOAM ROLLING AND SELF-MYOFASCIAL RELEASE TECHNIQUES

Once the body is warmed up and the core temperature is elevated, athletes may want to perform active self-myofascial release techniques utilizing a foam roller on both the agonist and antagonistic muscles active in sporting movements. If the athletes are performing acceleration or linear speed work, the glutes need to be firing maximally. With this knowledge, the athlete will perform myofascial release work for about 1-3 minutes on the hip flexors and surrounding hip musculature, then slowly sink into a stretch for these muscles for approximately 6-10 seconds per side. Three reps of this lengthening stretch per side should do the trick. After this stretching, isometric contraction of the glutes and/or dynamic contraction of the glutes can ensure proper firing of these powerful extensors of the hip.

Dynamic Warm-Up

DYNAMIC MOVEMENT PATTERNS

- 20yards form skipping down and back
- 20yards jogging down and back
- 20 yards high knees
- 20 yards butt kickers
- 20 yards back pedaling down and back
- 20 yards carioca down and back facing same direction
- 20 yards tin man
- 20 yards external/internal hip rotations
- 20 yards power skipping
- 20 yards skater hops
- 20 yards bear crawl
- 20 yards zig zag ¾ sprints
- 20 yards 90% effort sprint

DYNAMIC STRETCHES

- 10-15 Forward backward inside leg pendulum swings
- 10-15 Forward backward butt kicker leg pendulum swings
- 10-15 side to side leg pendulum swings
- 10-15 lateral upper body rotations
- 10-15 lower upper body rotations
- 10-15 high upper body rotations
- 10-15 lateral arm swings
- 10-15 up down arm swings
- 10-15 waiter arm swings
- 10-15 shoulder rotations front and back
- 10-15 neck rotations
- 10s hand and foot shakes

NEUROMUSCULAR WARM UP EXERCISES

- Body Squats
- Step Forward Lunges
- Jump Squats
- Split Squats
- Agility Ladder
- 4 Points Supermans
- Inchworm
- 4 point Hip Exercises
- Burpees
- Plank Rotations
- Low Back Extensions

CHAPTER IX

IN-SEASON PROGRAMMING FOR SPORT

In-Season Football Programming

After a grueling off-season consisting of intense weight room workouts, agility and speed training, skill work, position specific drills, and game-play, many football players often end their summers in optimal physical condition. From gains in strength, power, and hypertrophy to enhanced speed and agility, these results are usually a testament to how hard these athletes have worked in the off-season.

Off-season strength and conditioning has become a year round part of the game. The weight room is a part of football, with improvements in this area oftentimes leading to improvements on the field. Quite common is the fact that the athletes with the best strength and power relative to their body weight are often those seeing the most time on the field.

In season training for football is an often overlooked component of the game. Whether due to time commitments, energy levels or just a lack of knowledge of the importance of this aspect of training, once the season begins, oftentimes, the off-field training ends.

Through proper off season training, including optimizing muscular balance, a football player can make vast improvement in their on-field markers for performance. For instance, with increases in lower extremity muscular balance, an athlete may see greater flexibility in their hips, leading to greater efficiency in gluteal, adductor and hamstring muscle fiber activation. With this increase in glute and hamstring, hip extensor strength/activation, an athlete may experience an increase in on-field acceleration.

Understanding that football is a sport that consists of short burst acceleratory and power movements, with moderate rest in between repetitions, the importance of maintaining strength and power becomes even more apparent. Maintaining those hard earned results is crucial for success all season long.

Football by the Numbers:

Variable	Average Result
Average length of a play	4s [1]
Average Rest Period between plays	25-35s
Average Actual Time Ball is in Play (NFL)	10 minutes 43 seconds [1]
Work to Rest Ratio	1:10 [1]
Average 1RM Back Squat College	199.4kg (+/-51.8) [2]
Average Vertical Jump College	64.8cm (+/-2.9) [2]
Average 40 Yard Dash College	4.98s (+/-.31) [2]
Average % Bodyfat	13.2% (+/-3.5) [2]

Common Muscular Imbalances In Football

Shoulder Girdle Imbalances

Correcting muscular imbalances in the upper body, in particular the shoulder girdle musculature, should be high priority for football players. If the shoulders are rounded forward, there may be an imbalance between the pectoral musculature, lats, and the external rotator/mid trapezius/rhomboid musculature. With this internally rotated shoulder posture an athlete may be susceptible to shoulder injuries, especially while hitting or being hit by an opponent on the football field.

If the imbalance is corrected through targeted off and in-season training, the integrity of the shoulder capsule may be returned. With optimal shoulder stability the athlete may notice gains in the ability to generate force during impacts as well as increases in the weight room.

Quarterbacks in particular need to pay close attention to their muscular balance, as they not only require the ability to run, cut, avoid defenders, and absorb impacts, but they also need to throw. With this collection of skills, it is important for the quarterback to maintain optimum muscular balance. For example, if the shoulder girdle lacks the previously mentioned muscular balance between the external rotators/mid trapezius musculature and the pectoral/lat musculature, the athlete may exhibit an internally rotated humerus combined with rounded shoulders. This posture may impede throwing mechanics and decrease technical proficiency, potentially leading to an increase in chronic or acute injury.

By restoring the antagonistic muscle balance of an athlete's shoulder girdle and maintaining optimum muscular balance in the lower body, a quarterback can become a two-way threat on the field.

Corrective Exercise Recommendations

- Prone W, Y, T, L

- Incline Bench 2 arm Trap 3 Lift

- Dumbbell or Cable External Rotator Exercises

- Wall Dowel Rod Series

VMO Weakness

The VMO is a critical muscle for knee stability. Without optimal strength or activation of this muscle, actions such as cutting with cleats on, and tackling can leave the knee susceptible to injury. Along with this increased potential for injury, speed may be compromised as the VMO plays a considerable role in the final stages of knee extension. This is critical for the propulsive force required for sprinting and acceleration.

Corrective Exercise Recommendations

- Peterson Step Ups

- 1 ¼ dumbbell squats with heels elevated on incline board

- Split Squats

- Backward Sled Dragging

- Deep Front Squats

- Deep Back Squats

Weak Hamstrings as flexors of the knee

Due to lack of off-season training emphasis, many football players can develop knee stability issues due to weakness in the hamstrings as flexors of the knee. Most off-season programming consists of compound movements including squats, cleans, deadlifts, bench press, etc. If the hamstrings as flexors of the knee are trained directly, it is typically done via Swiss ball hamstring curls.

The hamstrings as flexors of the knee are also trained during sprinting movements, both through acceleration as well as deceleration of the lower leg. For many this may suffice, but for some, strength training is required. In particular unilateral strength training aimed at correcting muscular imbalances. Coach Charles Poliquin teaches the use of varied foot positions as well as use of different implements including standing, kneeling, prone, and seated hamstring curls.

Because of their insertion points, the hamstrings as flexors of the knee are important in football as these muscles help to stabilize the knee. With greater knee stability not only is injury potential minimized, but the ability to generate more force both on the field and in the weight room is realized.

Corrective Exercise Recommendations

- Kneeling Hamstring Curls

- Unilateral Prone Hamstring Curls

- Unilateral Seated Hamstring Curls

- Unilateral Swiss Ball Hamstring Curls

- Unilateral Standing Hamstring Curls

Inactivity of the Hip Extensor musculature

As many high school or college age football players sit in classrooms for hours on end during the day, their hip flexors may become shortened or tight. This can lead to a phenomenon known as reciprocal inhibition. With reciprocal inhibition, the nervous system responds by inhibiting the signal to the opposite muscles. In this case the hip extensors can become inhibited, particularly the glutes. Not only will athletes lose the ability to pull the ground behind them during sprinting and acceleratory movements, but they will also increase the potential for low back overuse injury and hip pain/injury.

Corrective Exercise Recommendations

- Glute Activation Exercises

- Full Squats

- Split Squat Variations

- Lunge Variations

- Deadlifts

- Romanian Deadlifts

- Sprinting

- Forward Sled Dragging

In-Season Football Programming

Sample 2 Day Per Week Hypertrophy Total Body Program

Day 1

Exercise	Rep Range	Sets	Tempo	Rest Interval
A1: Deadlift	6-8	3	3010	60s
A2: Flat Barbell Bench Press	6-8	3	3010	60s
B1: Back Squats	6-8	2	3010	60s
B2: Chin ups	6-8	2	3010	60s
C: Y,T,L	10,10,10	2	2010	45s

Day 2

Exercise	Rep Range	Sets	Tempo	Rest Interval
A1: Front Squat	5-6	3	3010	60s
A2: Pullups	8-10	2	3010	60s
B1: Dumbbell Split Squats	8-10	2	3010	60s
B2: Incline Dumbbell Bench Press	8-10	2	3010	60s
C: Seated Dumbbell External Rotator	10-12	2	2010	45s

In-Season Football Programming

Sample 2 Day Per Week Strength/Power Total Body Program

Day 1:

Exercise	Rep Range	Sets	Tempo	Rest Interval
A: Power Clean from mid thigh	2-3	3	X0X0	180s
B1: Back Squat	3-5	3	2010	90s
B2: Kneeling Hamstring Curls	4-6	3	3010	90s
C1: Close Neutral Grip Chins	3-5	3	2010	90s
C2: Incline Dumbbell Bench Press	3-5	3	2010	90s

Day 2:

Exercise	Rep Range	Sets	Tempo	Rest Interval
A1: Power Snatch from mid thigh	2-3	3	X0X0	180s
B1: Romanian Deadlift	3-5	3	2010	90s
B2: Flat Barbell Bench Press	3-5	3	2010	90s
C1: GHR	4-6	3	3010	90s
C2: Pullups	3-5	3	2010	90s

In-Season Soccer Programming

Known as one of the most popular sport in the world, soccer requires great degrees of coordination, speed, agility, lower body strength, and stamina. As a sport that consists of short burst sprints interspersed between periods of standing, walking and jogging, the energy system demands are both anaerobic and aerobic.

When preparing for a soccer season, many athletes overlook the importance of strength training, instead choosing to focus their efforts on long, slow endurance training and agility ladder or cone drills. This oversight can not only open the door to injuries, but can also lead to decreased performance on the field, as the athlete may lack anaerobic capacity and strength.

Another important element of off and in-season soccer training is upper body and lower back/core strength. In order to protect the ball or knock an opponent off the ball, there is physical contact. The combination of strong legs and a strong low back/core will enable an athlete to maintain upright stability when engaging an opponent. Upper body strength is important for throw-ins, fighting for position during corner kicks, running speed, and fending off the opposition.

In order to avoid the pitfalls of in-season performance deterioration, it is critical not to overlook these elements during off-season training. Soccer athletes should seek to improve upon each of these during the season, while enhancing individual skills and overall team play.

Soccer by the Numbers

Variable	Average Result
Average High Intensity Sprint	3.7-4.4s [2]
Average Distance Of High Intensity Sprint	24.5yds [2]
Average Recovery Between Sprints	40-70s [2]
Percentage Of Activity Spent Standing	4.6% [1]
Percentage Of Activity Spent Walking	14.2% [1]
Percentage Of Activity Spent Jogging	28.1% [1]
Percentage Of Activity Spent Running	11.1% [1]
Percentage Of Activity Spent Shuffling	9.3% [1]
Percentage Of Activity Spent Skipping	9.9% [1]
Percentage Of Activity Spent Sprinting	4.8% [1]
Percentage Of Activity Spent Other	18.1% [1]

Common Muscular Imbalances In Soccer

Hip Flexor Tightness (plant leg vs. kicking leg)

Many soccer players can develop a pelvic shift and rotation due to the nature of their sport. As they plant their leg to strike the ball during the kicking motion, they initiate a powerful hip flexion followed by knee extension and pelvic rotation. This series of movements done over a lifetime can lead to a pelvic imbalance from the tightening of the kicking leg hip flexor and internal rotation of the plant leg. The imbalance may appear as a pelvic hike toward one side, a rotated pelvis, or a pelvic tilt. It may also appear as a combination of any one of these. This may also lead to imbalances in the low back musculature.

Corrective Exercise Recommendations

- Split Squats

- Overhead Squats

- Hip flexor stretching

- Bridges

- Windshield Wipers

- Swiss Ball Stir the Pot

VMO Weakness

A combination of tight hip flexors and lateral quadriceps dominance can potentially increase susceptibility for knee injury. Oftentimes when using the overhead squat to evaluate an athlete with the combination of a pelvic imbalance and tight hip flexors/lateral quad dominance, valgus knee stress, excessive torso lean, and internal rotation of the heels results. An athlete with weakness of the VMO may have difficulty stabilizing the knee medially. This lack of medial stabilization and the resultant internal rotation of the femur may leave the knee more susceptible to injury.

Corrective Exercise Recommendations

- Peterson Step Ups

- Split Squat Variations

- 1 ¼ dumbbell squat variations

- Heels elevated squat variations

- Backward sled drag variations

Weak Core musculature

Weakness of the muscles about the core can lead to a dramatic decrease in the quality of movement. Many soccer players commonly perform horizontal based core strengthening exercises as a part of their strength and conditioning preparation. These exercises are great for improving movement quality, enhancing core strength/activation, and rehabbing or correcting muscular imbalances and movement dysfunctions. The problem lies in the fact that these exercises are the only core exercises many soccer players use for core strengthening.

The core consists of the muscles in the front and back directly above and directly below the pelvis. These muscles are responsible for stabilization of the body during static positions and dynamic movement, in all postures. Most team sports consist primarily of movements in standing positions, but yet, most core exercises performed by soccer players are in either supine or prone positions.

After they have learned to engage their core properly and have increased strength and movement quality from horizontal positions, athletes need to progress to upright core exercises. These will teach and strengthen the bracing mechanism that creates upright stability during both static and dynamic movements.

Corrective Exercise Recommendations

- Swiss Ball Stir the Pot:

- Rotational Plank:

- Overhead Squat:

- Asymmetrical Loading:

- Chin ups:

- Modified Strongman Training:

- Counter Rotation Exercises:

Upper Body Weakness

As a majority of the sport consists of lower body movements, soccer players often overlook the value of upper body strength training. A strong upper body can not only be of tremendous benefit in keeping an opponent off the ball, but it can also aid in position for corner kicks and throw ins. Emphasizing quality upper body strength training can oftentimes give the soccer player the much needed edge on the field of play.

Corrective Exercise Recommendations

See Programs below

In-Season Soccer Programming

Sample 2 Day Per Week Hypertrophy Split Program

Day 1: Upper Body

Exercise	Rep Range	Sets	Tempo	Rest Interval
A1: Chin Ups	8-10	2	3011	60s
A2: Flat Dumbbell Bench Press	8-10	2	3010	60s
B1: 1 Arm Dumbbell Rows	10-12	2	3011	60s
B2: Standing Dumbbell Overhead Press	10-12	2	3011	60s
C1: Standing Cable External Rotator	10-12	2	3010	45s
C2: Single Arm Trap-3 Lift	10-12	2	2010	45s

Day 2: Lower Body

Exercise	Rep Range	Sets	Tempo	Rest Interval
A1: Deadlift	6-8	2	3010	60s
B1: Dumbbell Split Squats	8-10	2	3010	60s
B2: Box Step Ups	8-10	2	1010	60s
C1: Low Back Extensions	8-10	2	3011	60s
C2: Reverse Hyperextensions	8-10	2	3011	60s

In-Season Soccer Programming

2 Day Per Week Strength/Power Split Program

Day 1: Legs

Exercise	Rep Range	Sets	Tempo	Rest Interval
A: Power Clean from mid thigh	2-3	3	X0X0	120s
B: Back Squat	4-6	3	3010	90s
B2: Hamstring Curls	3-5	3	3011	90s
C: Dumbbell Split Squats	5-7	2	3010	90s

Day 2: Upper Body

Exercise	Rep Range	Sets	Tempo	Rest Interval
A1: Push Press	3-5	3	20X0	120s
A2: Pullups	4-6	3	3011	90s
B1: Flat Dumbbell Bench Press	3-5	2	3010	90s
B2: 1 Arm Dumbbell Row	4-6	2	3010	90s
B3: Single Arm Trap-3 Lift	6-8	3	3010	90s

In-Season Baseball Programming

As a sport dominated by explosive movements separated by long periods of rest, baseball requires the ability to go from 0 to 60 repeatedly throughout the course of a game. During the season, athletes should seek to maintain or increase rotational power, pitching/throwing velocity, acceleration, and agility through proper training of their fast twitch muscle fibers.

Powerful activation of the legs, hip rotators, spinal musculature, shoulders and wrist are all required for success in baseball. These explosive movements combined with structural imbalances can oftentimes increase the potential for injury. For example, baseball player swinging a bat in the same direction an average of 250 times per week, accumulates 1000 swings per month and roughly 12,000 swings per year. When done over a career, this can lead to an over-development of rotational muscles on one side of the body, and underdevelopment of the rotary muscles on the other side. Unless these imbalances are addressed, this can result in back pain, hip problems, or a torque posture.

Baseball by the Numbers

Variable	Average Result
Average Sprint Duration To First Base	5.03s [1]
Times Per Game Sprint To First Base	2.4 times per game [1]
Average Duration Between Pitches	21.6s [1]

Common Muscular Imbalances In Baseball

Rotator Cuff Weakness

Due to the range of motion combined with tremendous arm velocity, pitching can put tremendous amounts of stress on the elbow and entire shoulder complex, in particular, the muscles of the rotator cuff. If left unchecked, these forces can increase the potential for injury about these joints. This stress becomes even more of a hazard when the athlete is in a state of fatigue.

To minimize the potential for injury about the rotator cuff and shoulder, a wide variety of rotator cuff exercises and drills needs to be utilized in order to strengthen the muscles that stabilize the shoulder.

Corrective Exercise Recommendations

- Seated Dumbbell External Rotator:
- Wall Dowel Rod Shoulder Series:
- Standing Cable External Rotator
- Shoulder Horn Dumbbell External Rotator
- Elbow Supported External Rotator
- W, Y, T, L
- Cable Scap Retraction:
- Trap 3 Lift

Low Back and Core Strength

Strong low back and core musculature allow for increased stability and rotational power in an upright position. For example, with weakness in the muscles that connect the torso to the pelvis, baseball players may risk injury to the back due to an increase in the stress placed upon the sacroiliac joint. Not only will strengthening these muscles keep the risk of injury to a minimum, but it will also help in enhancing speed, acceleration, stabilization, and generation of rotational power.

Corrective Exercise Recommendations

- Kneeling Landmine
- Rotary Cable Work
- Counter Rotation Exercises
- Rotational Plank:
- Farmer Carry

- Asymmetrical Loading

Rotational Movement Energy Leaks

When evaluating a baseball player, having them perform a rotational med ball throw can provide insight into various energy leaks or disconnect through the kinetic chain. For example, a right handed batter with a weak VMO on the right side may demonstrate a break in the ground reaction force transfer up the kinetic chain. This break may occur as an inward collapsing of the knee, leading to a decrease in the rotary hip mechanics. With this decreased power coming from the hips, greater demand is placed on the low back, obliques, and shoulder to complete the movement powerfully.

Keeping the entire kinetic chain strong from point of impulse on the ground up through the entire chain until the ball leaves the arm or bat is critical.

Corrective Exercise Recommendations

VMO Strengthening:

- Peterson Step Ups:
- Backward Sled Drags:

Rotary Strength:

- Windshield Wipers
- Lateral Med ball Counter Rotation Exercises:
- Pallof Press:
- Rotational Low Back Extensions:
- Kneeling or Standing Landmine:

Lateral Hip Strengthening:

- Lateral Band Walks
- Lateral Sled Drags
- Asymmetric Loading Exercises:

Shoulder Strengthening:

- Kneeling Cable Scarecrows

- Band Pull Aparts

- Scap Rows

- T's

In-Season Baseball Programming

2 Day Per Week Hypertrophy Total Body Program

Day 1

Exercise	Rep Range	Sets	Tempo	Rest Interval
A1: Dumbbell Squats	6-8	3	3010	60s
A2: Standing Dumbbell Overhead Press	8-10	3	3010	60s
B1: Dumbbell Split Squats	6-8	2	3010	60s
B2: Neutral Grip Chin Ups	8-10	2	3010	60s
C: Y,T,L	10,10,10	2	2010	45s

Day 2

Exercise	Rep Range	Sets	Tempo	Rest Interval
A1: Deadlift	6-8	2	3010	60s
A2: Flat Dumbbell Bench Press	8-10	2	3010	60s
B1: Step Forward Lunges	6-8	2	3010	60s
B2: Inverted Rows	8-10	2	3010	60s
C1: Seated Dumbbell External Rotator	10-12	2	2010	45s
C2: Trap-3 Lift	10-12	2	2010	45s

In-Season Baseball Programming

2 Day Per Week Strength/Power Split Program

Day 1: Legs

Exercise	Rep Range	Sets	Tempo	Rest Interval
A: Clean High Pull from mid thigh	2-3	3	X0X0	120s
B1: Back Squats	4-6	3	3010	90s
B2: Prone Lying Hamstring Curls	3-5	3	3011	90s
C: Rotational Back Extensions	8-10	2	3010	90s

Day 2: Upper Body

Exercise	Rep Range	Sets	Tempo	Rest Interval
A1: Push Press	3-5	3	20X0	120s
A2: Neutral Grip Chin ups	4-6	3	3011	90s
B1: Flat Dumbbell Bench Press	3-5	3	3010	90s
B2: 1 Arm Dumbbell Row	4-6	3	3010	90s
B3: Single Arm Trap-3 Lift	6-8	3	3010	90s

In-Season Hockey Programming

Tremendous emphasis is placed on off-season preparation in the sport of hockey. Many athletes realize the importance of being bigger faster and stronger. In the college weight room, many a division one hockey player could rival the physical prowess of their same size football counterparts.

Looking at the professional level, it becomes quite evident just how important strength and conditioning to the game. Hockey players have sought out quality strength coaches for years in hopes of extending their careers and enhancing their on ice performances. Many with great success.

As a sport that requires tremendous leg power and strength not only to stay upright on the skates, but also to generate enough force to propel the athlete down the ice, hockey is unparalleled in its demands for strength and stamina. Also important are structural strength and stability of the low back, core, and shoulder strength/stability for absorbing impacts and checking. Lactic acid clearance and buffering are also critical, as athletes are often pushing their bodies for over 45 second per shift.

The ability to control the puck is another critical element of the game. Whether it be bringing the puck up the ice while maintaining head up and vision forward/peripheral or shooting the puck accurately, the ability to maintain balance while evading defenders are just some of the elements that separate hockey from other sports.

Hockey By the Numbers

Variable	Average Result
Size of The Playing Surface	200ft X 11ft (North America), 210X98 (Eur)
Time Length of Game	60m
Average Length Of Shift	61s [1]
Average Shifts Per Period	5.2 [1]
Work To Rest Ratio	1:3.5-1:8 [3]

Common Muscular Imbalances In Hockey

Lateral Quadriceps Dominance/Medial Quadriceps Weakness

Hockey athletes are often lateral quadriceps musculature dominant due to the nature of the skating motion. With this lateral quadriceps dominance comes a medial quadriceps weakness, particularly in the Vastus Medialis Oblique. The VMO is a knee stabilizing muscle, playing a key role in medial/lateral tracking of the knee.

Corrective Exercise Recommendations

- Peterson Step Ups

- 1 ¼ dumbbell squats with heels elevated on incline board

- Backward sled dragging

Hamstring as flexor of the knee weakness

The mechanics of the skating motion require very little activation of the hamstrings as flexors of the knee. Compared to sports that require sprinting where the hamstring is used to accelerate the body as well as decelerate the lower leg, the skating motion has very little recruitment of the hamstrings as flexors of the knee. Due to the gliding motion in hockey, emphasis is placed on the quadriceps, hip flexors, and hip extensor musculature.

With their insertion points, the hamstrings as flexors of the knee are important in hockey as these muscles help to stabilize the knee. With greater knee stability not only is injury potential minimized, but the ability to generate more force both on the ice and in the weight room is realized.

Corrective Exercise Recommendations

- Single Leg Hamstring Curl Variations (kneeling, standing, seated, prone)

- Single Leg Swiss Ball Hamstring Curls

- Glute Ham Raise

Inactivity of the Hip Extensor musculature

With the rigidity of the skate and the inability of the foot to plantar flex and more importantly dorsiflex, the hip extensors may become inactive in certain ranges of motion. Take for example the squat exercise. The deeper you squat, the greater the glute, hamstring, and adductor recruitment. In order to squat to a low depth, dorsiflexion is required. World renowned fascial tissue and rehabilitation expert Chad Robertson has expressed that if the ability to dorsiflex is minimized, as is the case when wearing a rigid hockey skate, proper depth cannot be reached in the squatting exercise, which can then lead to minimized recruitment of the hip extensor musculature [2]. This weakness in the hip extensors can often lead to low back problems as well as hip pain.

Corrective Exercise Recommendations

- Full squats

- Split Squat variations

- Lunge Variations

- Deadlifts

- Romanian Deadlifts

- Sprinting

- Forward Sled Dragging

Low Back Imbalances

Upon taking thousands of slap shots from one side or the other over a lifetime of playing hockey, imbalances throughout the low back musculature may occur. Oftentimes when evaluating the low back muscle hypertrophy and strength levels of a hockey player, greater hypertrophy can be seen on one side of the spinal erectors vs. the other. This is often combined with lateral deviations during back extension testing exercises.

Corrective Exercise Recommendations

- Side Plank Holds

- Planks with Rotation

- Side lying raises

- Rotational Low back extensions

- Palloff Press

- PNF Cable Lifts

- Standing Single Arm Cable Rows

Muscular Imbalances about the Shoulder Girdle

Skating down the boards, looking to dump the puck off, and suddenly the athlete is blindsided with a punishing check into the boards. The impact drives the athlete's shoulder directly into the boards, where it then crumples, fracturing the clavicle bone, dislocating the shoulder, and stretching the rotator cuff musculature and labrum. The athlete is left cringing in pain down on the ice, with their season potentially over.

Oftentimes there may be no way to prevent this perfect hit or the damage suffered from it, but there may be ways to minimize the impact on the shoulder.

If the shoulders are rounded forward due to excessive pull from the internal rotators including pectorals and lats, combined with weakness of the external rotators and scap retractors, the shoulder may be left in a position for potential harm. If the shoulders are pulled back and down due to a balanced pull between the antagonistic muscles, the shoulder complex may then become more stable, with greater potential for protecting against the impact that was seen during the check into the boards.

Corrective Exercise Recommendations

- Prone W, Y, T, L

- Incline Bench 2 arm Trap 3 Lift

- Dumbbell or Cable External Rotator Exercises

- Wall dowel rod series

In-Season Hockey Programming

2 Day Per Week Hypertrophy Total Body Program

Day 1

Exercise	Rep Range	Sets	Tempo	Rest Interval
A1: Deadlift	6-8	3	3010	60s
A2: Wide Neutral Grip Chinups	6-8	3	3010	60s
B1: Front Squats	5-6	2	4010	60s
B2: Flat Barbell Bench Press	6-8	2	3010	60s
C: Y,T,L	10,10,10	2	2010	45s

Day 2

Exercise	Rep Range	Sets	Tempo	Rest Interval
A1: Back Squat	6-8	3	3010	60s
A2: Incline Dumbbell Bench Press	6-8	3	3010	60s
B1: Dumbell Split Squats	6-8	2	3010	60s
B2: Bent Over Barbell Rows	6-8	2	3010	60s
C: Cuban Press	10	2	2010	45s

In-Season Hockey Programming

2 Day Per Week Strength/Power Split Program

Day 1: Legs

Exercise	Rep Range	Sets	Tempo	Rest Interval
A: Power Clean from mid thigh	2-3	3	X0X0	180s
B: Back Squats	3-5	3	3010	90s
C1: Hamstring Curls	3-5	3	3011	90s
C2: Step Forward Lunges	4-6	3	3010	90s

Day 2: Upper Body

Exercise	Rep Range	Sets	Tempo	Rest Interval
A: Push Jerk	3-5	3	X0X0	180s
B1: Flat Dumbbell Bench Press	3-5	3	3110	90s
B2: Fat Grip Chin Ups	3-5	3	3010	90s
C2: Cuban Press	6-8	3	3010	90s

In-Season Basketball Programming

Basketball is a sport with many physical demands. Whether it be sprinting, jumping, boxing out, or lateral movement, an ability to perform all of these proficiently combined with great game skill can separate the bench players from the starting five. Endurance, both short burst interval and constant movement, are also critical elements of the game.

Regarding strength and conditioning, many basketball players emphasize the ability to jump higher. Entire books and programs are bought with the expectation of increasing an athlete's vertical jump. Focusing on strengthening of the hip extensors as primary muscles for increasing vertical jump can also carryover to an athlete's ability to accelerate and sprint.

One of the major issues with physical training for basketball is that weight training is often not emphasized until athletes reach the college level. For the youth athlete, weight training can be of benefit toward increasing vertical jump, acceleration, cutting ability, general physicality, and getting a leg up on the competition.

Basketball by the Numbers

Variable	Average Result
Court Size	94ft X 50ft (NBA), 84X50 High School
Game Duration	48 min (NBA), 40 min (College), 32 min (HS)
Average Distance Covered In Junior Elite Game	7558m [1]
Distance Covered Low Intensity Activity	2477m [1]
Distance Covered Moderate Intensity	1619m [1]
Distance Covered High Intensity	1743m [1]
% Of Time Above 95% Max HR	19.3 % [1]
% Of Time Between 85-95% Max HR	56% [1]
Average Duration Of Sprint	2.1s [2]
Average Duration Of Jump	1.0s [2]
Average Duration Of Run	2.3s [2]
Average Duration Of Jog	2.2s [2]
Average Duration Of Walk	2.4s [2]
Average Duration Of Standing	2.3s [2]

Common Muscular Imbalances In Basketball

Single Leg Dominance

In youth basketball, the simple footwork of learning to do a layup consist of a couple of dribbles, a large step onto the same side foot as the hand you are dribbling, then another large step onto the opposite foot, and jump as high as you can. Done over a lifetime, one leg may become much stronger than the other due to the repetition of the explosive jumping movement. This imbalance can often be seen in an athlete when they step under the squat rack. As they begin to descend, a weight shift may occur toward the dominant leg. The same may occur during the concentric contraction. Correcting this can not only enhance an athlete's ability to sprint and jump off of two feet, but it also may decrease the risk of injury.

Corrective Exercise Recommendations

- Peterson Step Ups

- Split Squats

- Lunge Variations

- Box Step Ups

- Asymmetric Loading Exercises

- Single leg sub maximal plyometrics

VMO Weakness

Possibly due to the lateral dominant movements such as cutting and defensive drills, or just a lack of proper training, a weak VMO muscle in basketball players can increase the potential for injury and potentially decrease jumping ability. As the VMO is highly active in the end ranges of knee extension, it plays a critical role in the final push off the ground in the jumping motion. If basketball athletes wish to ensure they are not limiting their jumping potential, strengthening of the VMO in a standing position needs to be a priority.

Corrective Exercise Recommendations

- Farmer Carry

- Peterson Step Ups

- 1 ¼ Dumbbell squats with heels elevated

- Backward Sled Drags

Achilles Tendon Tightness

In many, dehydration, weakness of the calf musculature, muscular imbalance between calf and tibialis musculature, and overuse of the Achilles tendon can lead to pain, tightness or tear in the tendon. Many vertical jump programs put an emphasis on high repetition calf training to enhance vertical jumping. Understanding the fact that the calves are only about 9-15% of an athlete's jumping power, wouldn't it make more sense to put the emphasis on lower rep calf training combined with powerful hip extensor training as these can account for as much as 60% of an athlete's jumping ability. Besides, this could also save the Achilles tendon from overuse.

Corrective Exercise Recommendations

- Electrolytes: Rehydrating

- Tibialis Anterior Training:

- Ankle Strengthening Exercises

Low Back Imbalances

Whether due to their long frames, inconsistent training habits, inflammatory diets, hip musculature imbalances, weak core muscles, obesity, structural issues, low testosterone, dehydration, weakness of the hip or low back musculature and more, basketball players have been known to have low back problems. Watching games back in the early nineties, I can remember seeing certain superstars lying face down on the floor to ease the pain in their low backs. Whatever the cause, correcting the problem should be a priority.

Corrective Exercise Recommendations

- Side Plank Holds

- Planks with Rotation

- Side lying raises

- Palloff Press

- PNF Cable Lifts

- Low Back Extensions

- Swiss Ball Stir the Pot

In-Season Basketball Programming

2 Day Per Week Hypertrophy Total Body Program

Day 1

Exercise	Rep Range	Sets	Tempo	Rest Interval
A1: Rack Pulls	5-7	3	3010	60s
A2: Flat Barbell Bench Press	6-8	3	3010	60s
B1: Step Forward Lunges	6-8/leg	2	2010	60s
B2: Chin ups	8-10	2	3010	60s
C: Y,T,L	10,10,10	2	2010	45s

Day 2

Exercise	Rep Range	Sets	Tempo	Rest Interval
A1: Box Squat	6-8	3	3010	60s
A2: Standing Dumbbell Overhead Press	8-10	3	3010	60s
B1: Dumbell Split Squats	6-8	2	3010	60s
B2: Pull ups	8-10	2	3010	60s
C: Cuban Press	8-10	2	2010	45s

In-Season Basketball Programming

2 Day Per Week Strength/Power Total Body Program

Day 1:

Exercise	Rep Range	Sets	Tempo	Rest Interval
A: Power Clean from mid thigh	2-3	3	X0X0	180s
B1: Push Jerk	3-5	2	2010	90s
B2: Step Forward Lunges	4-6/leg	2	2010	90s
C1: Close Neutral Grip Chins	3-5	2	2010	90s
C2: Romanian Deadlift	4-6	2	3010	90s

Day 2:

Exercise	Rep Range	Sets	Tempo	Rest Interval
A1: Power Snatch from mid thigh	2-3	3	X0X0	180s
B1: Box Squat	4-6	2	2010	90s
B2: Flat Barbell Bench Press	3-5	2	2010	90s
C1: Reverse Hyperextension	4-6	2	3010	90s
C2: Wide Pull ups	3-5	2	2010	90s

In-Season Field Hockey Programming

Field hockey is a sport that consists of both aerobic and anaerobic energy system demands. Whether sprinting, jogging, or walking, field hockey consists of the ability to control a solid plastic ball with roughly a 3 foot stick, while sprinting at near top speeds. From open field sprinting without the ball to rapid changes of direction and acceleration in small space, field hockey players need to possess both short burst and long sprint abilities.

Hand eye coordination also plays a key role in field hockey. In order to control the ball, especially during dynamic movement, field hockey players need to keep one eye on the ball, while maintaining their focus on the field of play. Another important element of field hockey is rotary power. In order to shoot and pass accurately without risk of injury, an athlete must possess optimal rotational power and flexibility.

Field Hockey by the Numbers

Variable	Average Result
Length Of Game	70 min
Length Of Field	91.4m X 55m
Average Duration Of Maximal Sprint	2s [1]
Percentage Of Activity Standing	5.8% [2]
Percentage Of Activity Walking	49.7% [2]
Percentage Of Activity Jogging	25.8% [2]
Percentage Of Activity Running	12.3% [2]
Percentage Of Activity Fast Running	4.9% [2]
Percentage Of Activity Sprinting	1.5% [2]

Common Muscular Imbalances In Field Hockey

Lateral Quadriceps Dominance/Medial Quadriceps Weakness

Field Hockey athletes can be lateral quadriceps musculature dominant due to the nature of the movements in their sport. With this lateral quadriceps dominance comes a medial quadriceps weakness, particularly in the Vastus Medialis Oblique. The VMO is a knee stabilizing muscle, responsible for control of medial/lateral tracking of the knee.

Corrective Exercise Recommendations

- Peterson Step Ups

- 1 ¼ dumbbell squats with heels elevated on incline board

- Backward sled dragging

Hamstring as flexor of the knee weakness

Due to the ratio of sprinting to lower intensity movement, the hamstrings as flexors of the knee may become weak. Because of their insertion points, the hamstrings as flexors of the knee are important in field hockey as these muscles also help to stabilize the knee. With greater knee stability not only is injury potential minimized, but the ability to accelerate and decelerate are enhanced.

Corrective Exercise Recommendations

- Single Leg Hamstring Curl Variations (kneeling, standing, seated, prone)

- Single Leg Swiss Ball Hamstring Curls

- Glute Ham Developer

Low Back Imbalances

Participation in any stick or racket based sport that requires rotational movements can leave the door open for muscular imbalances. Controlling the ball on the preferred side while in a bent over position can increase the potential for muscular imbalances throughout the low and mid back. Oftentimes when evaluating the low back muscle hypertrophy and strength levels of a field hockey player, greater hypertrophy can be seen on one side of the spinal erectors vs. the other. This is often combined with lateral deviations during back extension testing exercises.

Corrective Exercise Recommendations

- Side Plank Holds

- Planks with Rotation

- Side lying raises

- Rotational Low back extensions

- Palloff Press

- PNF Cable Lifts

- Standing Single Arm Cable Rows

In-Season Field Hockey Programming

2 Day Per Week Hypertrophy Total Body Program

Day 1

Exercise	Rep Range	Sets	Tempo	Rest Interval
A1: Dumbbell Deadlift	8-10	3	3010	60s
A2: Flat Dumbbell Bench Press	10-12	3	3010	60s
B1: Dumbbell Split Squats	8-10	2	3010	60s
B2: Neutral Grip Chinups	8-10	2	3010	60s
C: Y,T,L	10,10,10	2	2010	45s

Day 2

Exercise	Rep Range	Sets	Tempo	Rest Interval
A1: Dumbbell Squats	8-10	3	3010	60s
A2: Pushups	10-12	3	3010	60s
B1: Romanian Deadlifts	8-10	2	3010	60s
B2: 1 Arm Dumbbell Rows	10-12	2	3010	60s
C: Cuban Press	10	2	2010	45s

In-Season Field Hockey Programming

2 Day Per Week Strength/Power Total Body Program

Day 1:

Exercise	Rep Range	Sets	Tempo	Rest Interval
A: Power Clean from mid thigh	2-3	3	X0X0	180s
B1: Push Press	3-5	2	20X0	90s
B2: Back Squat	3-5	2	2010	90s
C1: GHR	4-6	2	2010	90s
C2: Close Neutral Grip Chins	3-5	2	2010	90s

Day 2:

Exercise	Rep Range	Sets	Tempo	Rest Interval
A1: Clean High Pull from mid thigh	2-3	3	X0X0	180s
B1: Front Squat	3-5	2	2010	90s
B2: Pullups	3-5	2	2010	90s
C1: Reverse Hyperextension	4-6	2	3010	90s
C2: Incline Dumbbell Bench Press	4-6	2	2010	90s

In-Season Lacrosse Programming

As a sport that requires a combination of stick handling skills, hand eye coordination, and conditioning, strength, speed, and power, Lacrosse is unique among field sports. At any time during a game, a lacrosse player may be required to sprint at maximal pace, cut on a dime, and/or absorb physical contact, all while maintaining possession of the ball.

Physiological characteristics can vary from position to position. Midfielders are required to perform longer sprint activities, while attack and defensemen require short burst explosive movements. Due to the nature of each position, demands of strength can also vary from position to position.

Lacrosse by the Numbers

Variable	Average Result
Length Of Game	15 min quarters (college), 12 min quarters (HS)
Size Of Lacrosse Field	110 X 60 yards
Average Distance Per Sprint	10-40 yards [1]
Average Time Between Sprints	5-15s [1]

Common Muscular Imbalances In Lacrosse

Rotator Cuff Weakness

An athlete whom demonstrates tight pecs/anterior deltoid musculature combined with weak external rotators/mid trapezius muscles may have an internal rotation about the shoulders, leading to a "Gorilla" like posture in their shoulders. Many therapists refer to this as upper cross syndrome.

To add insult to injury, the hundreds of shots and long passes the average lacrosse player practices per day can further exacerbate the issue. This dysfunctional posture may lead to a decrease in passing and shooting performance, as proper range of motion about the shoulder capsule is inhibited. It may also become more difficult for the athlete to increase or maintain the velocity of their shot while injury potentially can increase dramatically.

Corrective Exercise Recommendations

- 2 Arm Trap 3 Lift

- Wall Dowel Rod Shoulder Series

- Chin ups

- W,Y,T, L

- Single Arm Dumbbell Overhead Press

- Cable External Rotator Exercises

Low Back Imbalances

A strong low back allows for increased stability in an upright position. For example, without strong low back muscles connecting the torso to the pelvis, lacrosse athletes may not be able to absorb the impact of an opponent's cross check. Not only will a strong low back keep the risk of injury to a minimum, but it will also help in speed, acceleration, stabilization, and impact absorption.

Corrective Exercise Recommendations

- Deadlifts

- Modified Strongman Training

- Low Back Extensions

- Reverse Hyperextensions

- Side Plank

- Kneeling Landmine

- Windshield Wipers

In-Season Lacrosse Programming

2 Day Per Week Hypertrophy Split Program

Day 1: Upper Body

Exercise	Rep Range	Sets	Tempo	Rest Interval
A1: Flat Dumbbell Bench Press	8-10	2	3010	60s
A2: Wide Neutral Grip Chins	8-10	2	3010	60s
B1: Standing Dumbbell Overhead Press	10-12	2	3010	60s
B2: Bent Over Barbell Rows	10-12	2	3010	60s
C1: 2 Arm Trap 3 Lift	10-12	2	3011	45s
C2: Standing Cable External Rotator	10-12	2	2010	45s

Day 2: Lower Body

Exercise	Rep Range	Sets	Tempo	Rest Interval
A1: Front Squats	5-6	3	3110	60s
A2: Prone Hamstring Curls	6-8	3	3010	60s
B1: Romanian Deadlift	8-10	2	2010	60s
B2: Dumbell Split Squats	10-12	2	2010	60s

In-Season Lacrosse Programming

2 Day Per Week Strength/Power Total Body Program

Day 1:

Exercise	Rep Range	Sets	Tempo	Rest Interval
A: Power Clean from mid thigh	2-3	3	X0X0	180s
B: Push Jerk	3-5	2	20X0	90s
C1: Front Squat	3-5	2	2010	90s
C2: Kneeling Hamstring Curls	4-6	2	3010	90s
D1: Close Neutral Grip Chins	3-5	2	2010	90s
D2: Incline Dumbbell Bench Press	3-5	2	2010	90s

Day 2:

Exercise	Rep Range	Sets	Tempo	Rest Interval
A1: Power Snatch from mid thigh	2-3	3	X0X0	180s
B1: Back Squats	3-5	2	2010	90s
B2: Wide Pullups	3-5	2	2010	90s
C1: Reverse Hyperextension	4-6	2	3010	90s
C2: Dips	3-5	2	2010	90s

In- Season Rugby Programming

As a sport that consists of considerable strength, speed, and cardiovascular demand, rugby can be a difficult game to prepare for. Requiring both upper and lower body strength, short burst acceleration and 100m sprint ability, combined with the constant game play similar to that of soccer, the physical demands of Rugby fall across a very broad spectrum.

Rugby players today are bigger, faster, and stronger than their counterparts just 20 years ago. With a greater emphasis on strength and conditioning, the modern day Rugby athlete physique resembles more that of a football player rather than soccer athlete. On the professional level, it is not uncommon to see six foot plus athletes weighing over 230 pounds, with the ability to run the 100m near 11 seconds.

To perform effectively on the rugby field demands that all of the body's energy systems are developed to maximum levels. This can provide a serious challenge for players seeking to compete against the highest levels of competition. Maintaining and developing specific match fitness should be priority for any coach and players wishing to excel on the field.

Rugby by the Numbers

Variable	Average Result
Size Of Field Of Play	144m X 70m Max
Length Of Match	80 min
Ball In Play	33-36 min
Percentage Of Activity Spent Walking	Backs 38.7%/ Forwards 36% [1]
Percentage Of Activity Spent Jogging	Backs 27%/ Forwards 27.8% [1]
Percentage Of Activity Spent Cruising	Backs 9.3%/ Forwards 11.2% [1]
Percentage Of Activity Spent Striding	Backs 13.5%/ Forwards 15.15% [1]
Percentage Of Activity Spent Running	Backs 4%/ Forwards 5% [1]
Percentage Of Activity Spent Sprinting	Backs 7.2%/ 4.7% Forwards [1]
Average Distance Traveled In A Game: Backs	7225m [1]
Average Distance Traveled In A Game: Forw.	6677m [1]

Common Muscular Imbalances In Rugby

Knee Stability

As the VMO and hamstrings are critical muscles for knee stability, optimizing strength in these muscles should be a priority for the Rugby athlete. In the healthy knee, actions such as cutting with cleats on, tackling, and the open chaos of rucking and mauling can leave the knee susceptible to injury. Never mind the susceptibility of player exhibiting weak VMO and hamstrings as flexors of the knee. This athlete may have a tendency toward valgus stress (knock kneed) and knee instability, each of which can increase the potential for knee injury dramatically.

Corrective Exercises Recommendations

- Peterson Step Ups

- 1 ¼ dumbbell squats with heels elevated on incline board

- Backward sled dragging

- Hamstring Curls

- Hamstring Floor slides

- Deep Front Squats

- Deep Back Squats

Inactivity of the Hip Extensor musculature

As many Rugby players are either school aged athletes or working class people playing the sport they love, hip extensor activity may be compromised. Sitting down for hours on end during the day can lead to a shortening or tightening of the hip flexors. Once the hip flexors become shortened or tightened, they send a signal back to the brain telling it to shut down or minimize the activity of the opposite muscles, the hip extensors. In particular the glutes. This phenomenon is known as reciprocal inhibition.

With shortened hip flexors and inactive glutes as extensors of the hip, not only will athletes lose the ability to pull the ground behind them during sprinting and acceleratory movements, but they will also increase the potential for back injury and hip pain/injury.

Corrective Exercises:

- Glute Activation Exercises

- Full squats

- Split Squat variations

- Lunge Variations

- Deadlifts

- Romanian Deadlifts

- Sprinting

- Forward Sled Dragging

Low Back Imbalances

Whether it be job related, sport related, or just life related, we all have movement tendencies that can lead to muscular imbalances. These tendencies lead to repetitive motion, which can in turn lead to muscular imbalances. These then lead to compensations in movement. Tendencies may include preferring to cross on leg over the other, carrying a bag over one shoulder vs. the other, lifting things with one arm vs. the other and choosing to accelerate or decelerate more with one leg vs. the other. Over a lifetime, these imbalances can lead to decreases in the quality of athletic movements. Improving muscular balance throughout the low and mid back can aid in enhancing movement quality and efficiency.

Corrective Exercise Recommendations

- Side Plank Holds

- Planks with Rotation

- Side lying raises

- Asymmetric loading exercises

- Rotational Low back extensions

- Palloff Press

- PNF Cable Lifts

- Standing Single Arm Cable Rows

Muscle Imbalances about the Shoulder

Shoulder injuries can occur when a player with poor shoulder posture attempts to make an open field tackle. Especially in the sport of Rugby in which there is open field tackling with no pads to buffer the impacts. If the shoulders are rounded forward due to excessive pull from the internal rotators including pectorals, lats, combined with weakness of the external rotators and scap retractors, the shoulder may be left in a position for potential damage.

Corrective Exercise Recommendations

- Prone W, Y, T, L

- Incline Bench 2 arm Trap 3 Lift

- Dumbbell or Cable External Rotator Exercises

- Wall dowel rod series

In-Season Rugby Programming

2 Day Per Week Hypertrophy Total Body Program

Day 1:

Exercise	Rep Range	Sets	Tempo	Rest Interval
A1: Back Squats	6-8	3	3010	60s
A2: Chin Ups	6-8	3	3010	60s
B1: Rack Pulls	5-7	2	3010	60s
B2: Incline Dumbell Bench Press	6-8	2	3010	60s
C: Y,T,L	10,10,10	2	2010	45s

Day 2:

Exercise	Rep Range	Sets	Tempo	Rest Interval
A1: Front Squats	5-6	3	3010	60s
A2: Flat Dumbell Bench Press	6-8	3	3010	60s
B1: GHR	5-6	2	3010	60s
B2: Pull ups	6-8	2	3010	60s
C: Cuban Press	8-10	2	2010	45s

In-Season Rugby Programming

2 Day Per Week Strength/Power Total Body Program

Day 1:

Exercise	Rep Range	Sets	Tempo	Rest Interval
A: Power Clean from mid thigh	2-3	3	X0X0	120s
B1: Back Squat	3-5	3	2010	90s
B2: Incline Dumbbell Bench Press	4-6	3	3010	90s
C1: Barbell Front Rack Split Squats	4-6	3	2010	90s
C2: Neutral Grip Chin Ups	3-5	3	2010	90s

Day 2:

Exercise	Rep Range	Sets	Tempo	Rest Interval
A: Power Snatch from mid thigh	2-3	3	X0X0	30s
B1: Front Squat	3-5	3	2010	90s
B2: Flat Barbell Bench Press	3-5	3	2010	90s
C1: Romanian Deadlift	4-6	3	3010	90s
C2: Pullups	3-5	3	2010	90s

In-Season Softball Programming

Similar to baseball, softball is also a sport dominated by explosive movements separated by long periods of rest. Powerful activation of the legs, hip rotators, spinal musculature, shoulders and wrist are all required for success in many of the skills required of a good softball player. Whether it be underhand windmill pitching, batting, fielding, sprinting the bases, or throwing, softball players need to have a foundation of strength and stability in order to avoid injury.

Softball by the Numbers

Variable	Average Result
Duration Of Game	1.5-2.0 hrs
Distance To First Base	60 ft
Pitching Velocity (Rise ball 1996 Olympics)	97.2 km/hr [4]
Average Duration Between Pitches	17-18s (Olympic)
Expected Pitches Per Game (College)	Roughly 90 [1]
Max Bat Speed (Intermediate Level Player)	19 m/s [3]

Common Muscular Imbalances In Softball

Shoulder Problems

The 360-degree range of motion combined with tremendous arm velocity of underhand pitching can put tremendous amounts of stress on the rotator cuff muscles as well as the entire shoulder complex. This stress becomes even more of a hazard when the athlete is in a state of fatigue. To minimize the injury potential to the rotator cuff and shoulder, incorporating a wide variety of rotator cuff exercises can aid in strengthening the muscles that stabilize the shoulder girdle.

Corrective Exercise Recommendations

- Seated Dumbbell External Rotator

- Wall Dowel Rod Shoulder Series

- Standing Cable External Rotator

- Shoulder Horn Dumbbell External Rotator

- Elbow Supported External Rotator

- W, Y, T, L

- Cable Scap Retraction

- Trap 3 Lift

Low Back and Core Strength

Strong low back and core musculature allow for increased stability and rotational power in an upright position. Strengthening these muscles can help to keep the risk of injury to a minimum, as well as enhance bat speed, acceleration, stabilization, and rotational power generation.

Corrective Exercises:

- Kneeling Landmine

- Rotary Cable Work

- Counter Rotation Exercises

- Rotational Plank

- Farmer Carry

- Asymmetrical Loading

Unilateral Leg Dominance

The majority of the forces associated with hitting and pitching begin with the ground contact forces through the lower extremities. To throw with velocity and accuracy, pitchers require tremendous leg strength in both the push off and stride legs. Strength in the push off leg is required to transfer the ground reaction forces generated from the forward movement of the stride leg and arm. Conversely, the stride leg needs to be strong in order to absorb the eccentric forces associated with the pitching motion.

Likewise, leg strength and power are also important in hitting mechanics. The initiation of the movement begins with the ground contact forces traveling up through the back leg and hips, eventually resulting in a powerful weight shift and rotation of the pelvis and torso. From here the power is transferred through the upper extremities resulting in a powerful, fluid swing. It is for these reasons that unilateral leg training is imperative for avoiding muscular imbalances between right and left legs.

Corrective Exercise Recommendations

- Dumbbell Split Squats

- Lunge Variations

- Single-Leg Leg Press

- Sled Dragging

- Box Step Ups

Rotational Movement Energy Leaks

When evaluating a softball player, having them perform a rotational med ball throw can provide insight into various energy leaks or disconnect through the kinetic chain. For example, a right handed batter with a weak VMO on the right side may demonstrate a break in the ground reaction force transfer up the kinetic chain. This break may occur as an inward collapsing of the knee, leading to a decrease in the rotary hip mechanics. With this decreased power coming from the hips, greater demand is placed on the low back, obliques, and shoulder to complete the movement powerfully.

Corrective Exercise Recommendations

VMO Strengthening:

- Peterson Step Ups:

- Backward Sled Drags:

Rotational Strength:

- Windshield Wipers

- Lateral Med ball Counter Rotation Exercises:

- Pallof Press:

- Rotational Low Back Extensions:

- Kneeling or Standing Landmine:

Lateral Hip Strengthening:

- Lateral Band Walks

- Lateral Sled Drags

- Asymmetric Loading Exercises:

Shoulder Strengthening:

- Kneeling Cable Scarecrows

- Band Pull Aparts

- Scap Rows

- T's

In-Season Softball Programming

2 Day Per Week Hypertrophy Total Body Program

Day 1

Exercise	Rep Range	Sets	Tempo	Rest Interval
A1: Dumbbell Squats	8-10	2	3010	60s
A2: Standing Dumbbell Overhead Press	8-10	2	3010	60s
B1: Dumbbell Split Squats	8-10	2	3010	60s
B2: Neutral Grip Chin Ups	8-10	2	3010	60s
C: Y,T,L	10,10,10	2	2010	45s

Day 2

Exercise	Rep Range	Sets	Tempo	Rest Interval
A1: Dumbbell Deadlift	6-8	2	3010	60s
A2: Flat Dumbbell Bench Press	8-10	2	3010	60s
B1: Step Forward Lunges	8-10	2	3010	60s
B2: Inverted Ring Rows	8-10	2	3010	60s
C1: Standing Cable External Rotator	10-12	2	2010	45s
C2: Trap-3 Lift	10-12	2	2010	45s

In-Season Softball Programming

2 Day Per Week Strength/Power Total Body Program

Day 1:

Exercise	Rep Range	Sets	Tempo	Rest Interval
A1: Back Squat	3-5	2	2010	90s
A2: Standing Dumbbell Overhead Press	4-6	2	2010	90s
B1: Box Step Ups	5-7	2	1010	90s
B2: Neutral Grip Chin Ups	5-7	2	2010	90s
C1: Standing Cable External Rotator	6-8	2	2010	60s
C2: Single Arm Trap-3 Lift	6-8	2	2010	60s

Day 2:

Exercise	Rep Range	Sets	Tempo	Rest Interval
A1: Romanian Deadlift	4-6	2	2010	90s
A2: Flat Dumbbell Bench Press	4-6	2	2010	90s
B1: Dumbbell Split Squats	4-6	2	3010	90s
B2: Flat Dumbbell Bench Press	4-6	2	2010	90s
C1: Rotational Low Back Extensions	6-8	2	2010	60s
C2: Palloff Press	6-8	2	2010	60s

In-Season Golf Programming

Golf is a sport that consists of equal parts muscle control, power, and flexibility. As with any rotational sports that requires repetitive motion practice, muscular imbalances may occur. Injuries about the low back, knees, and elbows are common in golf.

Spinal path mechanics play an important role in golf. Due to the explosive rotational movements of the sport, participants lacking strength, flexibility, or movement quality may have increased potential for injury. Combine this with fatigue and faulty mechanics and the door opens for more serious injury.

With proper strength training protocols, athletes can develop optimal levels of strength, flexibility, muscle activation, and peripheral control.

Common Muscular Imbalances In Golf

Low Back Problems

The explosive rotational nature of the sport combined with the overloading of the swing pattern in one direction, imbalances about the low back can be prevalent amongst serious golfers. The athlete may be locked in rotation toward their dominant side. When examining the musculature of the low and mid back of a golfer, there are oftentimes visible differences between the spinal erectors on one side vs. the other. If these imbalances go uncorrected, not only is performance diminished over time, but the potential for hip structure imbalances and back strain is increased.

Corrective Exercise Recommendations

- Single arm Standing Cable Rows

- Kneeling Landmine

- Low Back Extensions with Rotation

- Rotational Plank

- 1 Arm Dumbbell Rows

- Suitcase Carries

Weakness of the rear leg VMO

Whether due to lack of training, past injuries, or poor swing mechanics, the vastus medialis oblique muscle on the inside of the back knee during the swing can often be weak in golfers. This weakness can lead to an increase in knee pain or increase the potential for more serious injury. As the VMO is a major stabilizer of knee tracking, strengthening this muscle can potentially enhance performance and decrease risk of injury.

Corrective Exercise Recommendations

- Peterson Step Ups

- Backward Sled Drags

- 1 ¼ Dumbbell Squats

- Heels Elevated Dumbbell Squats

Shoulder and Torso Rotational Mobility

One of the common complaints often heard from golfers is the lack of shoulder and rotational torso mobility. This is the mobility required to achieve full range of motion in both the swing and follow through.

Corrective Exercise Recommendations

- PNF Lift

- Wall Series

- Supine Rotational Torso Stretch

- Windshield Wipers

- Rotational Low Back Extensions

In-Season Golf Programming

2 Day Per Week Hypertrophy Split Program

Day 1: Upper Body

Exercise	Rep Range	Sets	Tempo	Rest Interval
A1: Lat Pulldowns	8-10	2	3010	60s
A2: Standing Dumbbell Overhead Press	8-10	2	3011	60s
B1: Seated Cable Rows	8-10	2	3011	60s
B2: Swiss Ball Dumbbell Bench Press	8-10	2	3010	60s
C1: Reverse PNF Chop	10-12	2	3010	60s
C2: Pallof Press	10-12	2	3011	60s

Day 2: Lower Body

Exercise	Rep Range	Sets	Tempo	Rest Interval
A1: Rotational Plank	8-10	2	3030	60s
A2: Supine Windshield Wipers	8-10	2	3030	60s
B1: Dumbbell Split Squats	6-8	2	2010	60s
B2: Swiss Ball Hamstring Curls	8-10	2	3010	60s
C1: Rotational Low Back Extensions	6-8	2	3011	60s
C2: Reverse Hyperextensions	8-10	2	3011	60s

In-Season Golf Programming

2 Day Per Week Strength/Power Split Program

Day 1: Legs

Exercise	Rep Range	Sets	Tempo	Rest Interval
A: Kettlebell Swings	12-15	3	X0X0	90s
B1: Dumbbell Squats	4-6	3	3010	90s
B2: Standing Hamstring Curls	3-5	3	3011	90s
C: Rotational Back Extensions	8-10	2	3010	90s

Day 2: Upper Body

Exercise	Rep Range	Sets	Tempo	Rest Interval
A1: Dumbbell Overhead Press	3-5	3	2010	90s
A2: Wide Grip Lat Pulldowns	4-6	3	3011	90s
B1: Flat Dumbbell Bench Press	3-5	3	3010	90s
B2: 1 Arm Dumbbell Row	4-6	3	3010	90s
B3: Single Arm Trap-3 Lift	6-8	3	3010	90s

In-Season Tennis Programming

Too often, young tennis players are pushed away from proper weight training and taught to focus more on ladder and hurdle speed, agility, and quickness training. Oftentimes this oversight results in aggravation of pre-existing structural imbalances and/or development of new ones.

The repetitive nature of the sport can lead to a wide spectrum of muscular imbalances in the tennis athlete. The explosive mechanics of serving can lead to shoulder and elbow issues. The biomechanical differences between backhand and forehand can lead to the over-development of low and mid-back musculature on one side versus the other. Along with improper backhand mechanics, weakness in the extensor carpi radialis muscle of the forearm can also be seen in those suffering from tennis elbow. Without correction, these imbalances can lead to decreased performance, chronic pain, and injury.

Repetitive trauma is often the culprit of many of the nagging injuries seen in tennis. When a movement pattern is repeated over and over again without proper strengthening of the antagonistic musculature, an overloading of those muscles and surrounding soft tissue can occur. The overloading of these muscles causes an imbalance between the prime movers (agonists), and the opposite muscles (antagonists). This overloading leads to a potential shortening and/or tightening of the prime movers and a stretching and/or lengthening of the antagonists.

Picture for a moment a bicep curl. The elbow flexors are the prime movers and the elbow extensors are the antagonists. If a trainee does only bicep curls for years on end without ever working their triceps, the elbow joint runs the risk of being locked in constant flexion due to the tightness of the biceps and weakness of the triceps.

For serious players, tennis is a year round sport. Keeping these athletes structurally balanced should be a priority. With practices nearly every day consisting of hundreds of strokes, serves, and volleys, the negative effects of overloading patterns can eventually creep in after years of training.

Overloading the same movement pattern over and over again can often lead to muscle imbalances. Just look at the shoulder of the hard serving tennis player who neglects proper shoulder strengthening.

What can be seen is a severe rounding forward or internal rotation of the serving shoulder due to thousands of repetitions over a career.

These imbalances can dramatically increase the potential for injury. Sitting in the stands while rehabbing an injury will not improve performance nor will it help the tennis athlete climb in the rankings. Muscular balance must be addressed through sound training practices.

Tennis by the Numbers

Variable	Average Result
Rest Between Points	20s (4)
Time Between Changeovers	90s (4)
Work To Rest Ratio	1:1-1:5 (4)
Total Playing Time	20-30% (1)
Average Length of a Point	3-15s (4)

Common Muscular Imbalances In Tennis

Internally Rotated Shoulder(s)

The biomechanics of a forehand and serve involve considerable amounts internal rotation. This overloading of the internal rotators can lead to a structural imbalance of the shoulder girdle, with the muscles responsible for external rotation potentially being exposed.

Both the muscles that externally rotate the humerus and the muscles that stabilize the scapula are important for maintaining shoulder stability. Just as baseball pitchers partake in extensive shoulder pre-habilitation, so too should tennis players seeking to improve upon performance and avoid potential shoulder injuries.

Corrective Exercise Recommendations

- Wall Series
- Cable External Rotator Variations
- Standing Cable Trap-3 Lift

Low back muscular imbalances

In tennis, and other rotary dominant sports, oftentimes structural imbalances can be seen in the torso, with the athlete locked into rotation toward their dominant side. When examining the musculature of the low and mid back of a tennis player, there can be visible differences between the low back musculature on one side vs. the other. If these imbalances go uncorrected, not only can performance diminished over time, but the potential for hip structure imbalances and back injury can be increased.

Corrective Exercise Recommendations

- Single arm Standing Cable Rows
- Kneeling Landmine
- Low Back Extensions with Rotation
- Side Plank

VMO Weakness

Activation and strength of the VMO muscle is critical for optimal knee stability. Responsible for regulation of knee tracking, the VMO is also an important muscle in the end ranges both knee flexion and knee extension. Keeping this muscle strong can aid in decreasing the potential for injury while increasing performance.

Corrective Exercise Recommendations

- Peterson Step Ups
- Backward Sled Dragging

Tight Hips

During the overhead squat evaluation, athletes may be unable to achieve full hamstring to calf squat depth due to hip flexor tightness and/or adductor tightness. With optimal hip mobility an athlete has a better chance of alleviating chronic back pains, increasing muscle activation of the hip extensor rotary musculature while decreasing the potential for injury. Increasing hip mobility can be done through stretching, strengthening, and/or both. One method of ensuring both is full-range of motion training.

Corrective Exercise Recommendations

- Split Squats

- Front Squats

- Split Squats

- Olympic Lifts

In-Season Tennis Programming

2 Day Per Week Strength/Power Total Body Program

Day 1:

Exercise	Rep Range	Sets	Tempo	Rest Interval
A1: PNF Reverse Chop	8-10	2	2010	90s
A2: PNF Chop	8-10	2	2010	90s
B1: Dumbbell Squat	5-7	2	2010	90s
B2: Standing Dumbbell Overhead Press	5-7	2	2010	90s
C1: GHR	5-7	2	2010	90s
C2: Neutral Grip Lat Pulldowns	5-7	2	2010	90s

Day 2:

Exercise	Rep Range	Sets	Tempo	Rest Interval
A1: Dumbbell Split Squat	5-7	2	2010	90s
A2: Flat Dumbell Bench Press	5-7	2	2010	90s
A3: Romanian Deadlift	5-7	2	2010	90s
A4: Seated Cable Rows	5-7	2	2010	90s
B1: Rotational Low Back Extensions	6-8	2	2010	60s
B2: Palloff Press	6-8	2	2010	60s

In-Season Volleyball Programming

As a sport that requires tremendous explosive power combined with linear and lateral agility, the demands of team volleyball are quite anaerobic in nature. When watching on television or in person, one can only marvel at the explosive athleticism of volleyball players, in particular the vertical jumping ability demonstrated during a kill or block. This combined with the hand eye coordination and quick burst acceleration required for digging and setting and it is easy to see why volleyball players need to emphasize strength and power during their physical preparation.

Another key element of volleyball is shoulder health. With the powerful spiking motion, there is potential for tightening of the muscles responsible for internal rotation and lengthening of the muscles responsible for external rotation. Keeping the muscles about the shoulder girdle strong and balanced can be a key not only greater success, but also career longevity

Volleyball by the Numbers

Variable	Average Result
Duration Of A Point	50% are 5-7s, 20% are 3s, 15% are 9-10s, 10% are > 15s [1]
Average Rest Between Points	12-14s [1]
Average Rallies Per Game	50 [1]
Average Rallies Per Five Game Match	250 [1]
Energy Systems	90% Anaerobic, 10% Aerobic

Common Muscular Imbalances In Volleyball

Internally Rotated Shoulder(s)

The biomechanics of the spiking and overhand serve motions require powerful internal rotation of the humerus. This overloading of the internal rotators can lead to a structural imbalance of the shoulder girdle, with the muscles responsible for external rotation becoming stretched, weak, and exposed.

Of particular importance are both the muscles that externally rotate the humerus as well as the muscles that retract and stabilize the scapula. Just as baseball pitchers undergo extensive shoulder pre-habilitation due to the repetitive mechanics of their sport, so too should volleyball players seeking to improve upon performance and avoid potential shoulder injuries.

Corrective Exercise Recommendations

- Wall Series
- Cable External Rotator Variations
- Seated Dumbbell External Rotator
- 2 Arm Trap 3 Lift
- Standing Cable Trap-3 Lift

Asymmetrical Imbalances of the Low Back

When examining the musculature of the low and mid back of a volleyball player, there may be visible differences between the low back muscles on one side vs. the other. If these imbalances go uncorrected, performance can be diminished over time due to energy leaks and decreased quality of movement. The potential for hip and back problems can increase as well.

Corrective Exercise Recommendations

- Single arm Standing Cable Rows
- Rotational Plank
- PNF Lift
- Kneeling Landmine
- Low Back Extensions with Rotation

VMO Weakness

Volleyball involves considerable amounts of lateral shuffling and quick burst sprints. The nature of these movements requires considerable lateral quadriceps muscle recruitment. This can create an imbalance between the lateral and medial quadriceps, in particular weakness of the VMO. Activation and strength of the VMO muscle is critical for optimal knee stability. Responsible for regulation of knee tracking, the VMO is also an important muscle in the end ranges of motion in both knee flexion and extension. Keeping this muscle strong can aid in decreasing the potential for knee injury while increasing jumping and acceleration potential.

Corrective Exercise Recommendations

- Peterson Step Ups

- Backward Sled Dragging

- Dumbbell Split Squats

- Front Squats

- Back Squats

- 1 ¼ Dumbbell Squats

- Heels Elevated Dumbbell Squats

In-Season Volleyball Programming

2 Day Per Week Hypertrophy Total Body Program

Day 1

Exercise	Rep Range	Sets	Tempo	Rest Interval
A1: Dumbbell Deadlift	6-8	3	3010	60s
A2: Incline Dumbbell Bench Press	8-10	3	3010	60s
B1: Dumbbell Split Squats	8-10	2	3010	60s
B2: Chinups	8-10	2	3010	60s
C: Y,T,L	10,10,10	2	2010	45s

Day 2

Exercise	Rep Range	Sets	Tempo	Rest Interval
A1: Dumbbell Squat	8-10	3	3010	60s
A2: 1 Arm Dumbbell Rows	8-10	3	3010	60s
B1: Step Forward Lunges	8-10	2	3010	60s
B2: Standing Dumbbell Overhead Press	8-10	2	3010	60s
C: Seated Dumbbell External Rotator	10-12	2	2010	45s

In-Season Volleyball Programming

2 Day Per Week Strength/Power Total Body Program

Day 1:

Exercise	Rep Range	Sets	Tempo	Rest Interval
A: Clean High Pull from mid thigh	2-3	3	X0X0	120s
B1: Split Squat	3-5	2	2010	90s
B2: Incline Dumbbell Bench Press	4-6	2	3010	90s
C1: GHR	3-5	2	2010	90s
C2: Wide Neutral Grip Chins	4-6	2	2010	90s

Day 2:

Exercise	Rep Range	Sets	Tempo	Rest Interval
A: Power Snatch from mid thigh	2-3	3	X0X0	120s
B1: Dumbbell Squat	3-5	2	2010	90s
B2: Standing Dumbbell Overhead Press	4-6	2	2010	90s
C1: Romanian Deadlift	3-5	2	3010	90s
C2: Kneeling Cable Scarecrows	8-10	2	2010	90s

In-Season Wrestling Programming

As gymnastics teaches an athlete to move and control their body in space, wrestling requires an innate ability to control and move an opponent's body in space. Physical elements including, takedowns and takedown defense, clinching, ground control, and escapes all require muscle endurance, metabolic conditioning, functional strength and last but not least, power.

Wrestlers often get into shape with minimal equipment by utilizing bodyweight circuits, kettlebells, sprinting and long distance endurance training, not to mention an abundance of live skill practice. All these play a critical role in the development of any grappling competitor.

Often overlooked though, is the development of true functional strength and power through sound training practices. In this case, the term functional strength can simply be classified as "usable" strength that can be easily transferred to increase one's ability in their sport. With a strong foundation of strength, an athlete can then increase their potential for increased rate of force development or power.

Wrestling by the Numbers

Variable	Average Result
Length Of A Match	3,2,2 min periods (College), three 2 min periods (HS)

Common Muscular Imbalances In Wrestling

Overuse Injuries

In preparing for season, many high school wrestlers participate in cross country with the hopes that long distance running will condition them for sport. One of the problems with this lies in the fact that when an athlete has faulty foot strike mechanics and they participate in long, slow, distance training, compensations and muscular imbalances can result.

With excessive endurance running, one of the imbalances that may result is lateral quadriceps dominance combined with lateral hip muscle imbalances. This can lead to lower extremity and hip problems including IT band inflammation, patellar tendonitis, shin splints, back problems, gluteal amnesia, lateral hip pain, and/or more.

Strengthening the body with corrective exercises and engaging in metabolic conditioning events that have a greater transfer of training effect is one strategy to minimize the overuse injuries associated with excessive slow distance running.

Corrective Exercise Recommendations

- Peterson Step Ups

- Split Squats

- Unilateral Hamstring Curls

- Glute Activation Series

- Reverse Hyperextensions

- Low Back Extensions

Low Back Imbalance

Many wrestlers have a dominant side to shoot with and well as perform throws with. Just like a laborer who carries lumber on his preferred shoulder for a lifetime, muscular imbalances throughout the back will appear. Oftentimes, there is much greater hypertrophy of the spinal erectors on the preferred side. When these athletes are asked to perform a low back extension, they often deviate or rotate toward the side with the greater hypertrophy, even though they think they are staying linear.

Corrective Exercise Recommendations

- Suitcase Carry

- Side Lying Raises

- Side Bridge

- Bird Dog

- Single Arm Cable Rows

Low Back Dominance Combined with hip extensor weakness

Athletes who have weak hip extensors yet strong low backs may complain of back pain. These athletes may be putting excessive demand on their low back musculature due to the fact that their hip extensors are either weak or not firing properly.

Corrective Exercise Recommendations

- Glute Activation Series

- Reverse Hyperextensions

- Romanian Deadlifts

- Kettlebell Swings

In-Season Wrestling Programming

2 Day Per Week Hypertrophy Total Body Program

Day 1

Exercise	Rep Range	Sets	Tempo	Rest Interval
A1: Deadlift	6-8	3	3010	60s
A2: Dips	8-10	3	3010	60s
B1: Back Squats	6-8	2	3010	60s
B2: Neutral Grip Chin Ups	8-10	2	3010	60s
C: Y,T,L	10,10,10	2	2010	45s

Day 2

Exercise	Rep Range	Sets	Tempo	Rest Interval
A1: Romanian Deadlift	6-8	3	3020	60s
A2: Flat Dumbbell Bench Press	8-10	3	3010	60s
B1: Dumbbell Split Squats	6-8	2	3010	60s
B2: Pullups	8-10	2	3010	60s
C: Seated Dumbbell External Rotator	10-12	2	2010	45s

In-Season Wrestling Programming

2 Day Per Week Strength/Power Total Body Program

Day 1:

Exercise	Rep Range	Sets	Tempo	Rest Interval
A: Clean High Pull from mid thigh	2-3	3	X0X0	120s
B1: Deadlift	3-5	2	2010	90s
B2: Standing Barbell Overhead Press	4-6	2	2010	90s
C1: GHR	3-5	2	2010	90s
C2: Neutral Grip Chin Ups	3-5	2	2010	90s

Day 2:

Exercise	Rep Range	Sets	Tempo	Rest Interval
A: Power Snatch from mid thigh	2-3	3	X0X0	120s
B1: Back Squat	3-5	2	2010	90s
B2: Flat Dumbell Bench Press	3-5	2	2010	90s
C1: Romanian Deadlift	4-6	2	2010	90s
C2: Wide Grip Pullups	4-6	2	2010	90s
D1: Rotational Low Back Extensions	6-8	1	2010	90s
D2: Standing External Rotator	6-8	1	2010	90s

CHAPTER X

EXERCISE TECHNIQUE

In any training program, technique and effort are two of the most important factors for success. Technique without effort can lead to little result, and likewise, effort with poor technique will yield less than desirable results. Learning technique through a book or video should in no way substitute for learning from an experienced strength coach or trainer.

In the realm of strength and conditioning, quite possibly the best technique for many exercises in this book can be taught by a Poliquin International Certified Professional. This is the certification created by the world's most successful strength coach, Charles Poliquin. Tapping into his three plus decades of experience as a world leader in the strength and conditioning industry, coach Poliquin has set the standard with his strength coach certification, with some of his students training the top athletes in many professional sports worldwide.

From Olympic weightlifting to structural balance training, to relative strength work to hypertrophy specific protocols, the methods and technique taught to PICP strength coaches are unparalleled. To learn more about the PICP coaching program or to find a PICP coach near you, check out www.charlespoliquin.com.

Other good sources of technical instruction are the United States Weightlifting Association (USAW), the NSCA CSCS, and Crossfit coaching courses. Though not the depth or extent of the PICP coaching course, each of these certifications does a good job in teaching athletes the basic strength and weightlifting technique necessary to achieve physical prowess on the field. To learn more about the USAW check out their website at www.weightlifting.teamusa.org. For more on the NSCA, their website is www.nsca-lift.com. Crossfit's main website is www.crossfit.com.

Back Squat

Classification: Lower body hip and knee extensor

Exercise Prerequisites: Glute, Hamstring, and Adductor activation. Avoid if chronic knee or low back pain.

Antagonistic Muscles to movement: Hamstrings as flexors of the knee.

Movement: Place hands on the bar slightly wider than shoulder width with thumbs and fingers around the bar. Rest the bar across the rear deltoids and upper trapezius, squeezing your shoulder blades down and together with chest out, making sure the bar does not rest across the lower neck or spine. Once you have un-racked the bar, assume a stable neutral/lordotic posture, keeping the weight balanced between feet, with equal distribution of throughout the foot. Place the feet hip width apart or slightly wider, with toes pointing straight ahead or slightly out. Keep your elbows pulled down. As you begin the descent, make sure to maintain lordotic posture beginning the decent by bending your knees first (a variation is to bend at the hips first). As you sit downward, begin pushing your knees outward to ensure maximum hip muscle recruitment. Once your hamstrings touch your calves, or you have gone as low as your flexibility allows, begin to initiate the ascent. Keeping the back arched/neutral with torso rigid, focus on driving the chest up first, keeping the torso upright.. Be sure to keep the heels driving into the ground, and avoid caving knees and rounding of the back. Make sure to exhale maximally after you have passed the sticking point and ascend all the way to the top. Then perform next repetition.

Keys to Movement:

1. Pinching shoulder blades back and down, rest bar across rear delts and upper trapezius.
2. Place feet hip width or slightly wider with toes pointing slightly outward.
3. Keep the elbows pulled downward.
4. Maintain neutral/lordotic posture while keeping the torso as upright as possible.
5. Bend at the knees first when you begin your ascent.
6. Push the knees outward, ensuring they point in the same direction as the toes throughout the movement.
7. Do not allow the heels to come off the ground or knees collapse throughout the movement.
8. Lower down until your hamstrings touch your calves or as low as your flexibility allows.
9. Initiate ascent by driving chest upward at first.

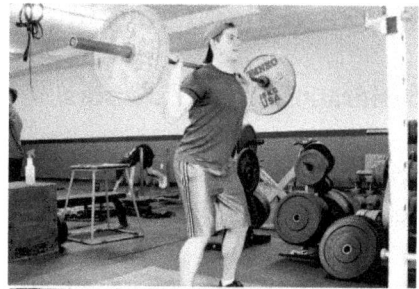

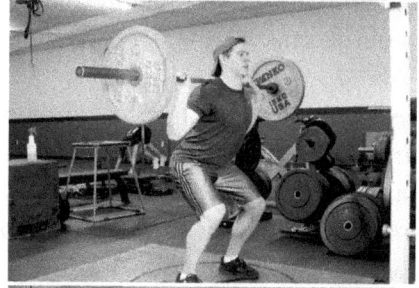

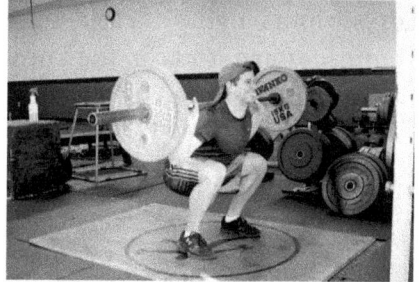

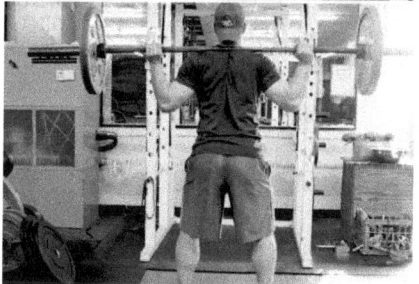

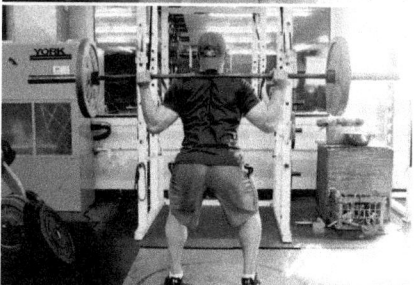

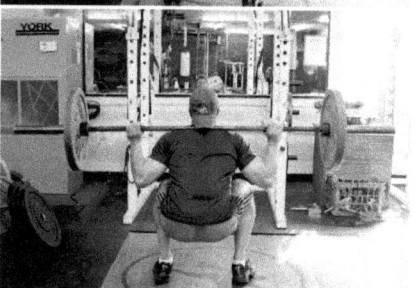

Backward Sled Dragging

Classification: Knee Extensors

Exercise Prerequisites: Avoid if you have persistent neck, knee, or low back pain.

Antagonistic Muscles to movement: Hamstrings as flexors of the knee.

Movement: Facing a sled while holding the handles, lean back with shoulders behind hips and feet hip width apart. Keeping hips extended and shoulders behind hips, begin walking backward focusing on fully extending the drive leg with each stride. Be sure not to reach back more than one foot length with the non-working leg as this can put unnecessary stress on the knee. The hips locked at 90 degrees sled drag as a viable option.

Keys to Movement:
1. Position feet hip width apart.
2. Lean back with hips extended and shoulders behind hips.
3. Focus on driving through the ball of the foot.
4. Extend the leg fully with each step.
5. Be careful not to step too far back and this can put excessive strain on the knee.

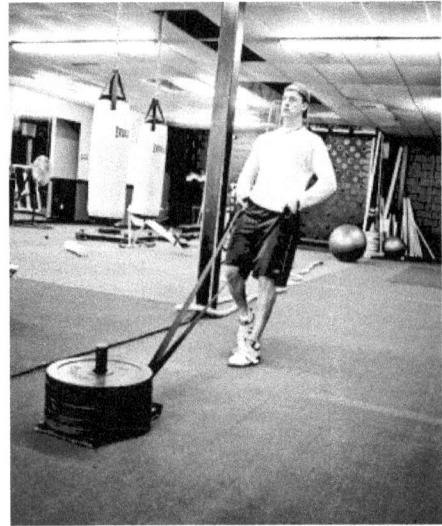

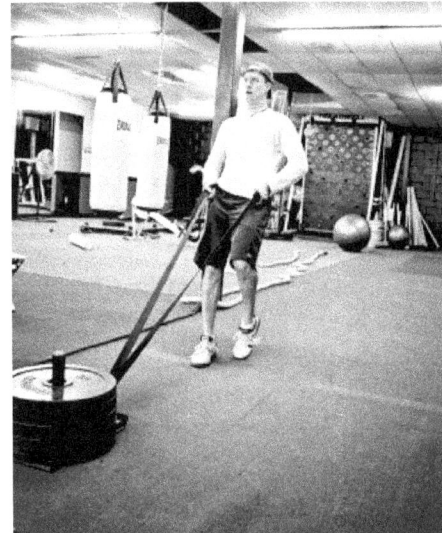

Barbell Bench Press

Classification: Upper Body Push

Target Muscles: Pectorals, Anterior Deltoids, Triceps

Exercise Prerequisites: Avoid exercise if you experience anterior or posterior shoulder pain, or AC joint pain. If upper crossed syndrome is an issue, perform corrective movements.

Antagonistic Muscles: Rhomboids, Trap 2-4, External Rotators

Movement: Lie on a flat bench with feet flat on the floor. Utilizing a pronated grip grasp the bar at bi-acromial grip, keeping the angle between the upper body and upper arm to 45 degrees or less. Pinch your shoulder blades back, hugging the bench, while expanding your chest upward.

Beginning with the barbell in the arms extended position, begin by lowering the bar straight down. Keep the upper arm angle relative to the body at 45 degrees or less.

Lower the bar down until it touches your chest. Without bouncing, keep the shoulder blades pulled back, begin the concentric action, retracing the same pattern the barbell was lowered. Breath out on the way up, while focusing on pectoral muscle recruitment.

Ensure the low back is pressed firmly against the bench to avoid neck or low back strain.

Keys to the Movement:
1. Grasp barbell with bi-acromial grip, hands in pronated position.
2. Upper arm at 45 degree angle or less relative to the upper body.
3. Keep low back firmly pressed against bench.
4. Pinch shoulder blades back with chest "out" to minimize shoulder injury potential.
5. Breath out during concentric movement.

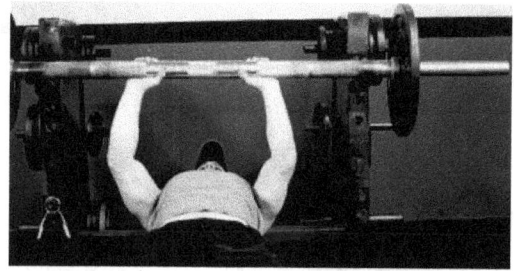

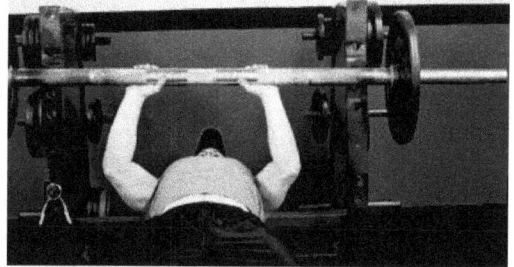

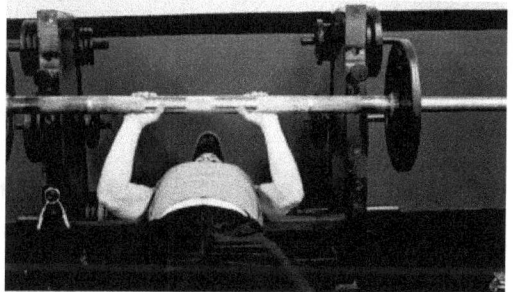

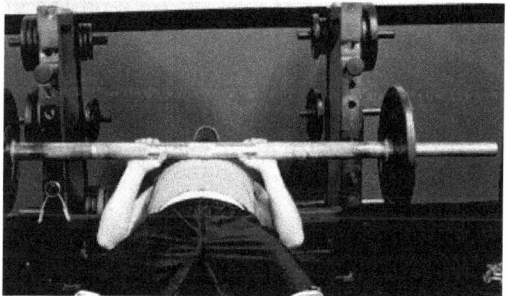

Barbell (Front Rack Position) Split Squat

Classification: Posterior Chain and knee Extensor

Exercise Prerequisites: Avoid if you have persistent neck, knee, or low back pain.

Antagonistic Muscles to movement: Hamstrings as flexors of the knee.

Movement: Position body with feet hip width apart, torso in neutral/slightly lordotic posture, with a barbell across your anterior deltoids and upper pectoral musculature. The "clean grip" is preferred. If you do not have the flexibility for the clean grip, use straps. Maintain upright posture throughout movement. With toes pointing straight ahead, step one foot forward into a lunge position. The distance between your feet is determined by your hip flexor range of motion. If the rear foot is too close, the heel of the front foot will come off during the movement. If the rear foot is too far back, the knee will not cross the heel plane. After you have found the optimal distance between front and rear foot, lower the hips forward and toward the ground maintaining upright posture with no lean forward in the torso. Keeping the back leg as straight as possible, descend until the hamstring comes in contact with the calf on the front leg. It is imperative not to lean forward or allow the front foot heel to come off the ground throughout the movement. As the hamstring comes in the contact with the calf, the knee may cross the toe plane. If the knees are healthy, this can help to strengthen the knee as there is a greater VMO, adductor, hamstring, and gluteal activation with deeper squats and lunges. Once the back knee is 1-2" above the ground initiate the backward movement through the ball of the front foot by driving the shoulders back to the start position with no change in posture. Make sure the front heel never comes off the ground or elevated platform. Perform all reps on one leg, then perform all reps on the opposite leg.

Keys to Movement:
1. Maintain lordotic/neutral posture with torso perpendicular to floor throughout the movement.
2. Determine optimal distance between front and rear foot.
3. Focus on keeping the back leg as straight as possible to ensure maximal tension on front leg and stretching of back leg hip flexor musculature.
4. Lower down until hamstring comes in contact with calf. In healthy knees, the knee may cross of the toe plane as there is a greater recruitment of VMO, adductor, hamstring, and gluteal musculature.
5. Begin ascent by focusing on driving the shoulders/torso back and upward first.
6. Do not allow the front heel to come off during the movement.
7. Do not allow torso to lean over during the movement.

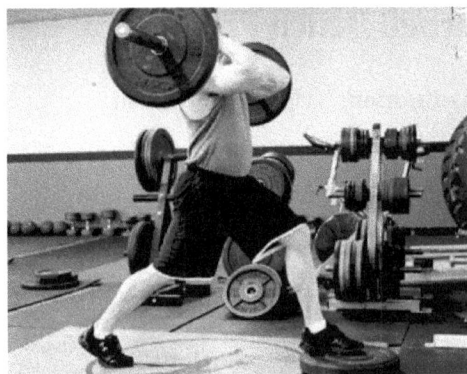

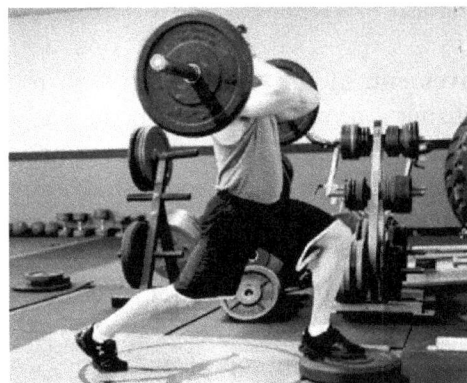

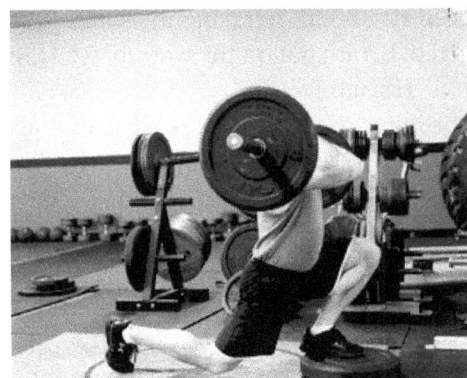

Bent Over Barbell Row

Classification: Upper Posterior Chain Pull Movement

Target Muscles: Trapezius, Latissimus Dorsi, Rhomboids, Rear Delts, Posterior Rotator Cuff Muscles, Low Back Extensor Chain, glutes, quads, hamstrings, tibialis anterior

Exercise Prerequisites: Correct activation of rear deltoids, rhomboids, and latissimus musculature. Avoid movement if you have low back pain

Antagonistic Muscles to movement: Shoulder internal rotators, elbow extensors.

Movement: Hold barbell in front of you with pronated grip and hands slightly wider than shoulder width. Bend your knees 20 degrees and lean over until your torso is parallel or near parallel to the floor. Arch your back into a lordotic posture, with chest out, shoulder pulled back and down, eyes straight down.

Maintaining torso parallel to the floor with lordotic posture, pull the weight toward your sternum/belly button, activating first the rear delt muscles, then pulling with the larger rhomboid and lat muscles. To do this, retract your shoulder blades back and down, then focus on pulling back with the elbows until full contraction of the upper back musculature.

Ensure not to allow the shoulders to shrug upward or come up, as this takes away from the contraction of the mid back/shoulder retractor muscles. Make sure there is no bounce or rounding of the back throughout the movement. Slowly lower the weight back to start and perform next repetition.

Keys to Movement:

1. Position body in correct starting position with knees bent 20 degrees, chest out, back arched, and torso parallel or near parallel to the floor.
2. Initiate movement by retracting shoulders back and down, maintaining torso posture.
3. Focus on pulling elbows back.
4. Do not allow shoulders to shrug upward.
5. Row back until complete contraction of shoulder blades.

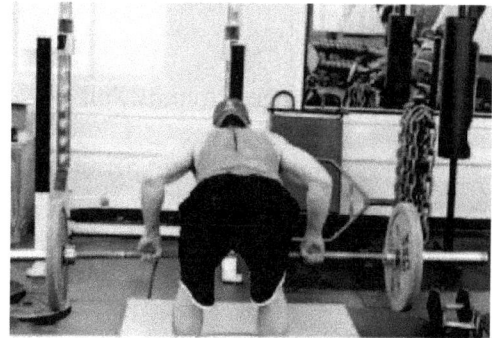

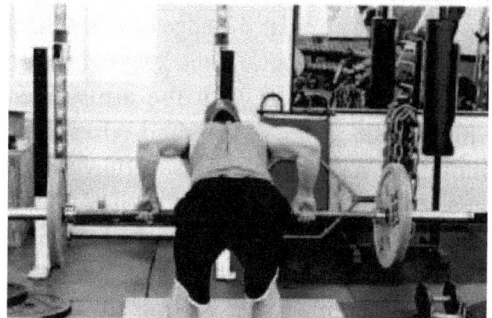

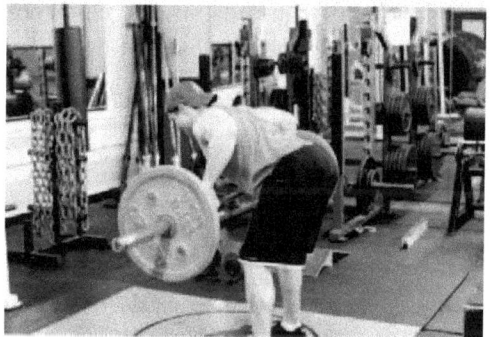

Bicep Curl

Classification: Upper Extremity Pull

Exercise Prerequisites: Do not perform if you have chronic shoulder, elbow, or neck problems.

Antagonistic Muscles to movement: Elbow Extensors

Movement: The seated version will allow for more isolation of movement. Sitting at the edge of a bench, retract the shoulder blades down and back while keeping the chin up and looking straight ahead. Start with the arms directly by your sides, with the pinky side of the hand offset closer to the end of the dumbbell. With palms up, arms fully extended, wrists straight or slightly extended, begin curling the weight upward. Be sure to disallow the upper part of the arm to move forward while raising the weight. During the entire range of motion, the shoulder blades are retracted and the head is looking straight ahead with the chin up. Once complete contraction has occurred, lower slowly back down to the full extension start position..

Keys to Movement:

1. Stand or sit with shoulder blades retracted and chest out.
2. Keep elbows at your sides.
3. Do not tuck your chin downward during the movement.
4. Focus on pulling with the pinky side of the hand.
5. Ensure complete range of motion by flexing the triceps at the bottom and flexing the biceps at the top of the range of motion.

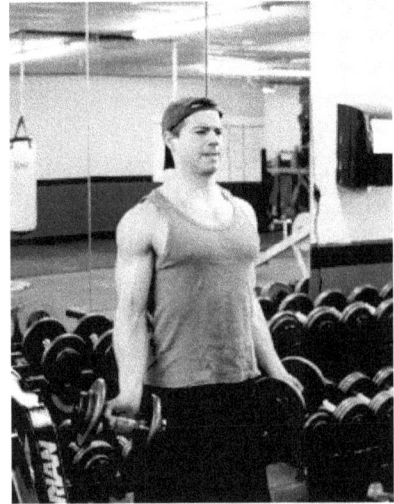

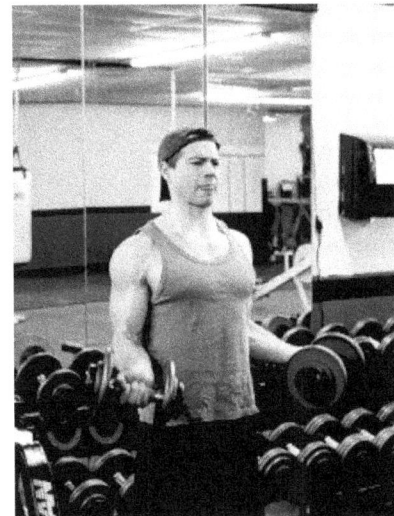

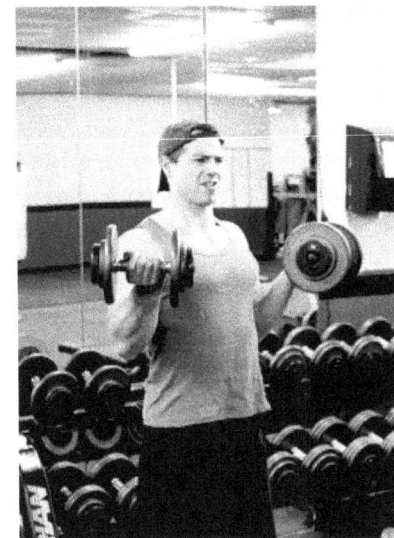

Box Jumps

Classification: Sub maximal Plyometric

Exercise Prerequisites: Avoid if you have chronic knee, ankle, or low back problems.

Movement: Standing erect in front of a box with your feet hip width apart and toes pointing forward. Rapidly bend at the knees, hips and ankles. Immediately reverse direction, extending knees, hip, and ankles and jump onto the box. Land quietly with feet hip width apart and knees pointing in the same direction as the toes. Ensure that you also minimize knee and hip flexion during the landing, allowing for no more than 90 degree flexion. Step off the box and perform next rep.

Keys to Movement:

1. Feet and knees pointing in the same direction during jump and landing.
2. Keep torso erect with neutral or lordotic posture throughout.
3. Land quietly with knee and hip flexion no greater than 90 degrees.

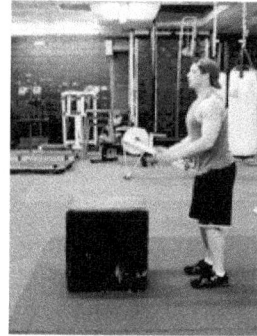

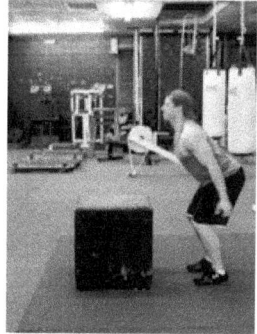

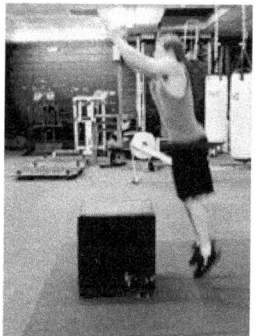

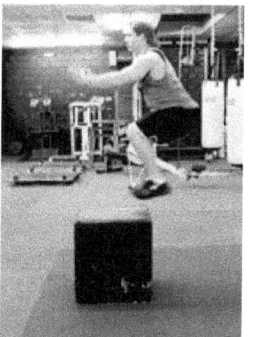

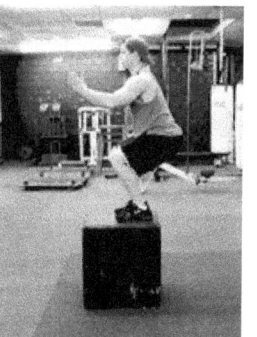

Box Step Ups

Classification: Posterior Chain Extensor

Exercise Prerequisites: Avoid this exercise if it aggravates knee, hip, or low back problems.

Movement: Choose a box height and stand with neutral posture beside the box. Step one foot up onto the box with the foot flat on the box and the other leg (foot on ground) in extended position, with foot fully plantar flexed or dorsiflexed and weight on the heels. Holding dumbbells down by your sides or a barbell across your shoulders, begin movement by driving chest and shoulders up first while minimizing assistance from foot on the ground.

Keeping your torso straight and perpendicular to the ground, focus on driving through the heel of the foot on the box, allowing for correct hip and knee extensor muscle activation.

Extend hip and knee of the drive leg until you have reached full extension of each joint. Do not allow the knee to collapse inward (valgus stress) during the movement.

Complete all reps on one leg and then perform reps on the other leg.

Keys to the movement:

1. Start with one foot on the box and the other on the floor in fully dorsiflexed or plantar flexed position with knee and hip extended.
2. Begin movement by driving chest and shoulders first, keeping torso perpendicular to the floor.
3. Without assistance from leg on the floor, extend hip and knee of leg on the box.
4. Do not allow the torso to lean or knee to collapse inward.

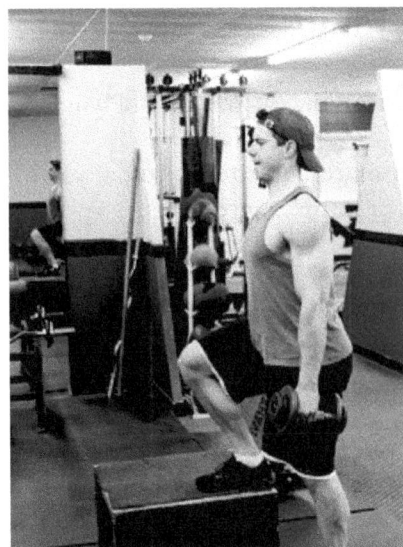

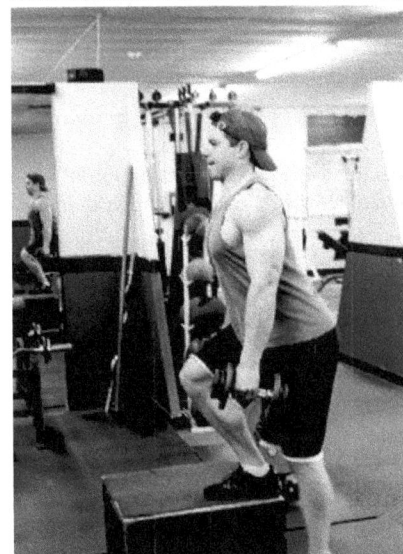

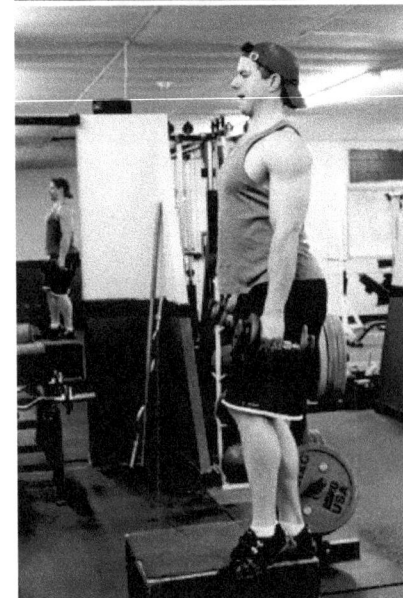

Chin-ups

Classification: Upper Posterior Chain Pull Movement

Target Muscles: Trapezius, Latissimus Dorsi, Rhomboids, Levator Scapulae, Brachialis, Biceps Brachii

Exercise Prerequisites: Correct activation of Latissimus Dorsi and rhomboids. Do not do if you have elbow, shoulder or serious low back pain

Antagonistic Muscles to movement: Internal rotators, elbow extensors

Movement: Grasp a pull-up bar with hands supinated, shoulder width or slightly wider. Hang from the bar, with arms, hips and shoulders in complete extension. Initiate movement by retracting shoulder blades back and down. Begin pulling your body straight upward, continuing to pull the shoulder blades back and downward. Do not allow the shoulder to internally rotate as you are pulling upward.

Pull upward, pinching your shoulder blades back until the upper portion of the chest comes in contact with the bar.

Lower the body slowly, retracing the same pattern until you reach full extension starting position at the bottom.

If you cannot perform a regular chin-up, you can use the assistance of a partner or a band around the knee or foot.

Keys to the Movement:

1. Supinated grip with hands shoulder width or slightly wider.
2. Begin in "dead hang" position.
3. Retract shoulders back and down prior to and during the movement.
4. Focus on pulling the elbows back and down.
5. Do not allow the shoulders to internally rotate,
6. Pull up until upper part of chest comes in contact with the bar.
7. Lower down until full extension in the elbows and shoulders.

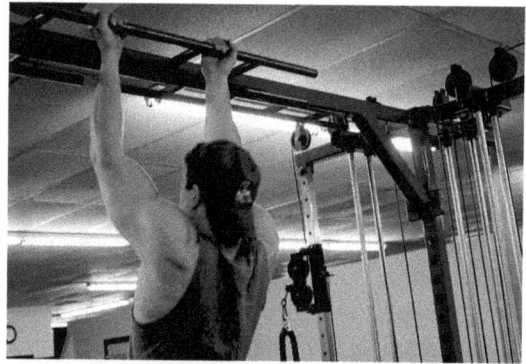

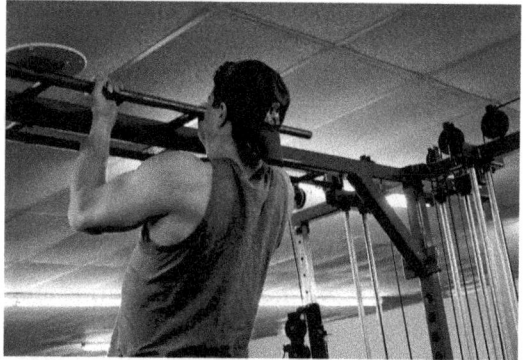

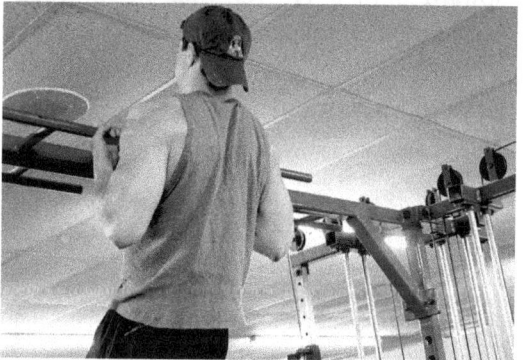

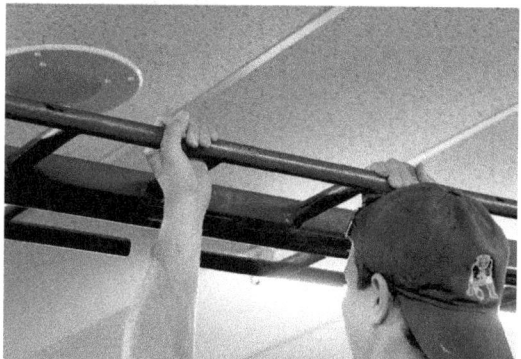

Cuban Press

Classification: Upper body press

Exercise Prerequisites: Avoid if you have persistent shoulder, neck, or low back pain.

Movement: Stand with feet hip width apart, holding a barbell or dumbbell with pronated grip. The width of the grip is determined by the length of your upper arms. Your grip width should be equal to the distance of both arms out to your sides with elbows bent 90 degrees and upper arm and forearms parallel to the floor. The width of your hands is the grip width you will take on the bar or dumbbells. The objective is to hold the elbows at 90 degree during the rotational component of the exercise.

Begin with arms extended and barbell roughly hip height. Begin by upright rowing the barbell, pulling the elbows as high as you can. Once the upper arms are out to your sides and parallel to the floor, externally rotate the forearms/barbell upward until it is over your head. Once over your head, overhead press the bar and lower back to start.

Keys to Movement:

1. Grip width is determined by the width of your upper arms out to your sides and 90 degree angle at the elbows. Ensure the upper arms and forearms are parallel to the floor when determining width.
2. Begin with barbell at roughly hip height.
3. Upright row the barbell, focusing on driving the elbows upward.
4. Once the upper arms are parallel to the floor, externally rotate the forearms/barbell until it is above your head.
5. Press overhead. Tuck the chin through as the barbell passes your forehead and focus on active shoulders at the top of the press.

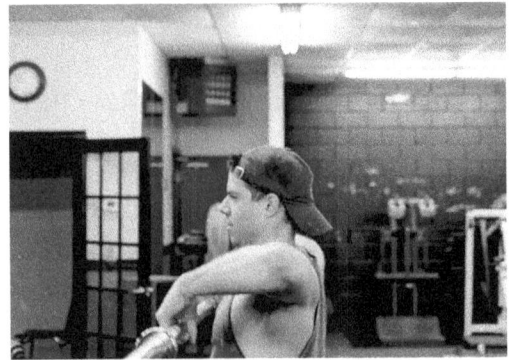

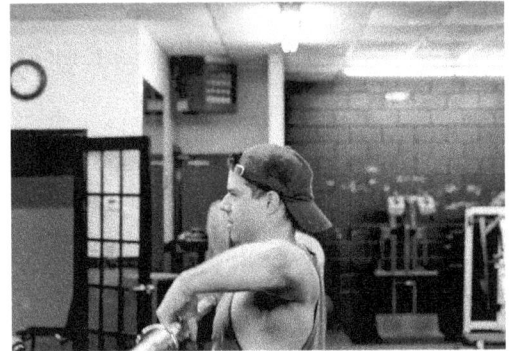

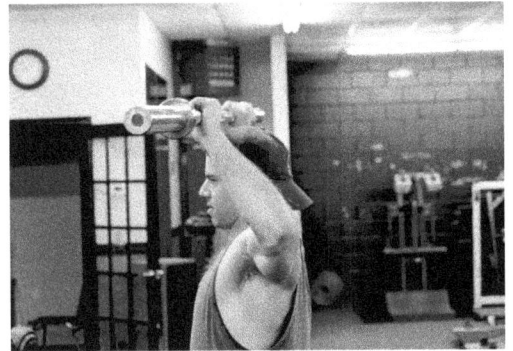

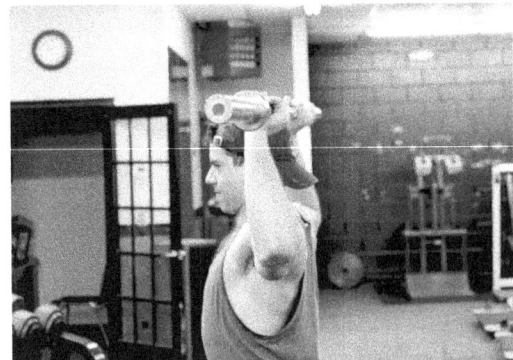

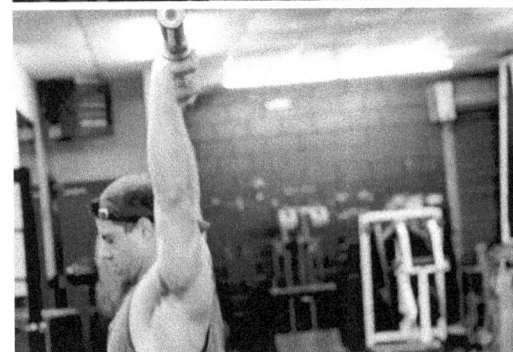

Deadlift

Classification: Posterior Chain Extensor

Exercise Prerequisites: Avoid if you have neck, knee, or low back pain or lack flexibility to assume proper starting position.

Movement: You can use an Olympic bar or a Hex deadlift bar. Pronated grip is preferred for higher repetitions while mixed grip may be preferred for lower reps. It is very important to begin the deadlift in the proper starting position as the mechanics and success of the movement depend heavily on this initial body positioning. Begin by creating a lordotic posture in the spine, with chest out, shoulder pulled back, eyes straight ahead. Lean the torso over to roughly 45 degrees and walk your shins to the bar or 1 inch away from the bar. Keeping the angle of the torso relative to the floor, begin bending at the knees in order to grasp the bar. Keep the weight shifted to the heels (you should be able to wiggle your toes in the start position). Once your body positioning is correct begin the lift by pulling the shoulders up first, trying to maintain torso angle and rigidity. Do not raise the hips first as this can put excessive strain on your low back ligaments. As you raise, focus on pulling the bar toward you, clearing your knees so the bar can travel in as straight a line as possible. Extend the hips and knees, increasing the torso angle, until the bar comes in contact with the bottom part of the upper thigh. Once you have reached complete extension of the hips and knees, retrace the movement pattern during the eccentric part of the movement.

Keys to movement:

1. Proper start position is imperative.
2. Roughly 45 degree of torso relative to ground.
3. Bar in contact with shins or one inch away in starting position.
4. Back arched with weight through the heels.
5. Mixed grip for low reps and pronated grip for higher reps.
6. Focus on raising the shoulders first, keeping the same angle at the torso throughout the movement.
7. Do not raise the hips first.
8. At the top of the movement, do not lean back.
9. Retrace the same movement pattern during the eccentric part of the movement.

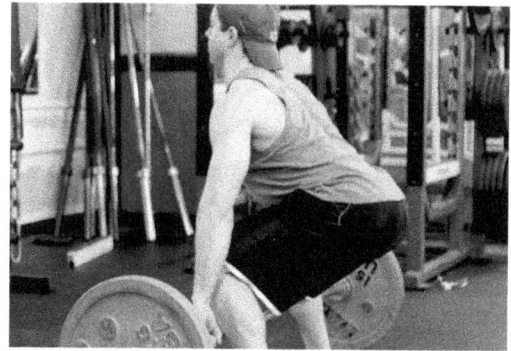

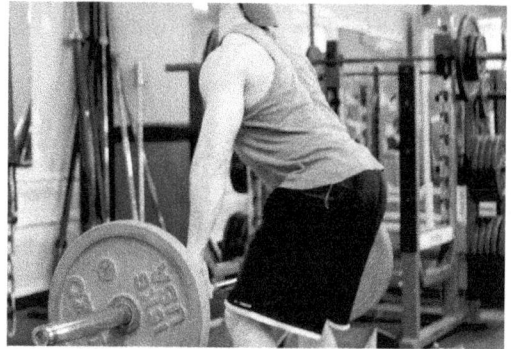

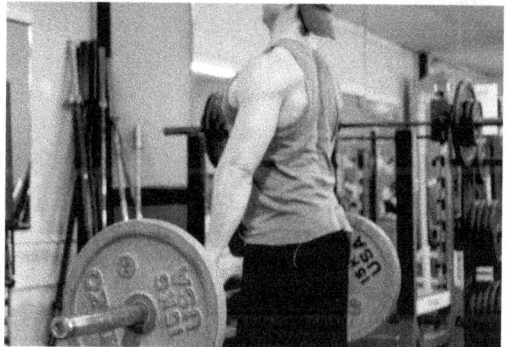

Dips

Classification: Upper Body Push

Target Muscles: Pectorals, Anterior Deltoids, Triceps

Exercise Prerequisites: Avoid exercise if you experience anterior or posterior shoulder pain, or AC joint pain. If upper crossed syndrome is an issue, perform corrective movements.

Antagonistic Muscles: Rhomboids, Trap 2-4, External Rotators

Movement: Start in the arms extended position with chest high, hips extended, and elbows pointing back. Begin lowering your body with your elbows pointing back or out to 45 degrees or less. Allow the body to lean slightly for greater pectoral recruitment. Lower until the brachioradialis makes contact with the bicep. Once at the bottom of the range of motion, begin concentric motion by focusing on driving the chest up first while keeping the elbows pointing back or out to 45 degrees or less. Press until arms are straightened and triceps are contracted.

In his book Target Bodybuilding, Author Per Tesch states "All three head of the triceps brachii are markedly used as you raise and lower the body."

In strength circles one of the best methods of improving the bench press in the structurally balanced trainee is to improve performance in dips. Other benefits of dips include minimal equipment requirements and maximal variation options. Dip variations include Gironda dips, elbow in, elbows out, isometric pauses at top of concentric or bottom of eccentric, torso perpendicular to the floor, torso slightly leaned forward, fat grip dips, and V bar dips.

Keys to the Movement:

1. Start with the eccentric contraction first
2. Begin with elbows pointing back or upper arms at 45 degree angle or less relative to the upper body.
3. Keep chest high.
4. Lower until biceps touch brachioradialis.
5. Initiate concentric motion by focusing on driving the chest up first.
6. End concentric motion once elbows are extended and triceps contracted.

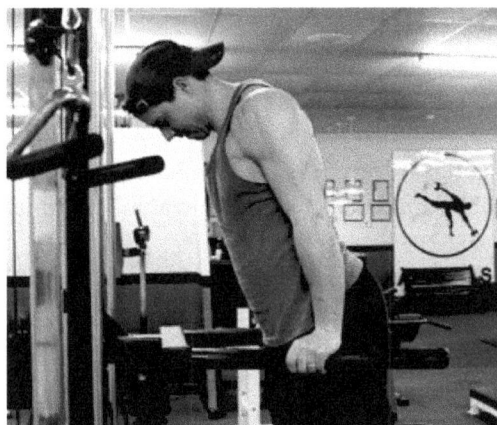

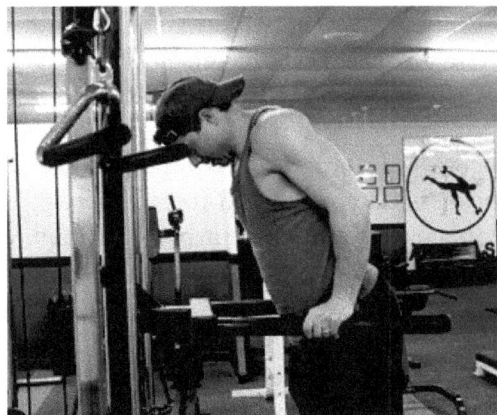

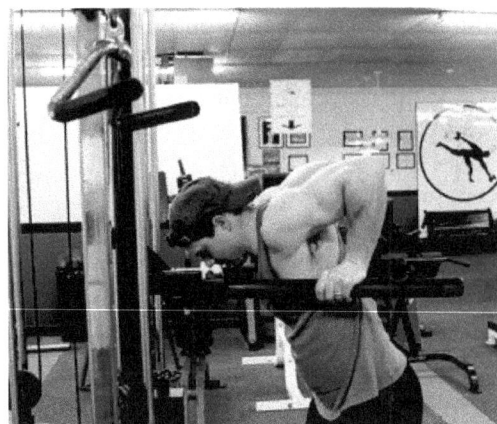

Drop Lunges

Classification: Posterior Chain and knee Extensor

Exercise Prerequisites: Avoid if you have persistent neck, knee, or low back pain.

Antagonistic Muscles to movement: Hamstrings as flexors of the knee.

Movement: Stand on a 4-6" elevated platform. Position body with feet hip width apart, torso in neutral/slightly lordotic posture, with dumbbells held at your sides or barbell across the shoulders or in font squat rack position. Maintain upright posture throughout movement. With toes pointing straight ahead, take a large step forward. Lower the hips forward and toward the ground maintaining upright posture with no lean forward. Keeping the back leg as straight as possible, descend until the hamstring comes in contact with the calf on the front leg. It is imperative not to lean forward or allow the front foot heel to come off the ground throughout the movement. As the hamstring comes in the contact with the calf, the knee may cross the toe plane. If the knees are healthy, this can help to strengthen the knee as there is a greater VMO, adductor, hamstring, and gluteal activation with deeper squats and lunges. Once the back knee is 1-2" above the ground initiate the backward movement through the ball of the front foot by driving the shoulders back to the start position with both feet on the platform with no change in posture. Perform all reps on one leg, then perform on the opposite leg.

Keys to Movement:

1. Stand on a 4-6" platform.
2. Maintain lordotic/neutral posture with torso perpendicular to floor throughout the movement.
3. Take a large step forward keeping the front heel in contact with the ground throughout the movement.
4. Focus on keeping the back leg as straight as possible to ensure maximal tension on front leg and stretching of back leg hip flexor musculature.
5. Lower down until hamstring comes in contact with calf. In healthy knees, the knee may cross of the toe plane as there is a greater recruitment of VMO, adductor, hamstring, and gluteal musculature.
6. Begin ascent by focusing on driving the shoulders/torso back and upward first.
7. Do not allow the front heel to come off during the movement.
8. Do not allow torso to lean over during the movement.

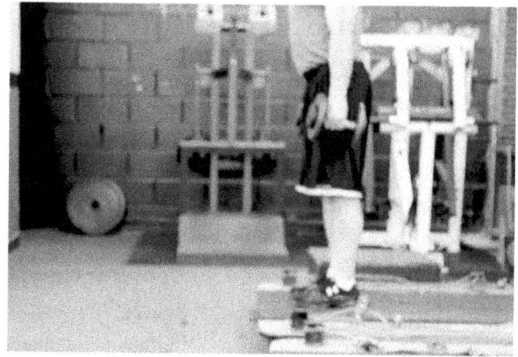

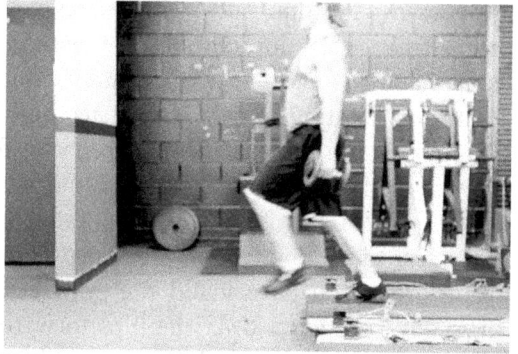

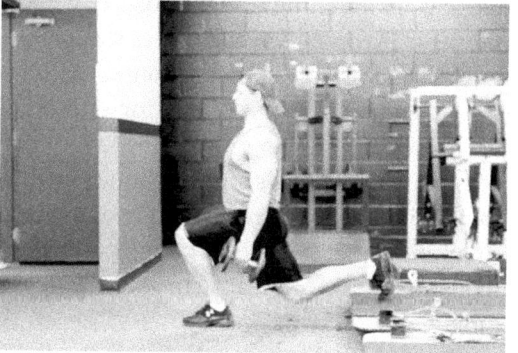

Dumbbell Split Squats

Classification: Posterior Chain and knee Extensor

Exercise Prerequisites: Avoid if you have persistent neck, knee, or low back pain.

Antagonistic Muscles to movement: Hamstrings as flexors of the knee.

Movement: Position body with feet hip width apart, torso in neutral/slightly lordotic posture, with dumbbells held at your sides. Maintain upright posture throughout movement. With toes pointing straight ahead, step one foot forward into a lunge position. The distance between your feet is determined by your hip flexor range of motion. If the rear foot is too close, the heel of the front foot will come off during the movement. If the rear foot is too far back, the knee will not cross the heel plane. After you have found the optimal distance between front and rear foot, lower the hips forward and toward the ground maintaining upright posture with no lean forward in the torso. Keeping the back leg as straight as possible, descend until the hamstring comes in contact with the calf on the front leg. It is imperative not to lean forward or allow the front foot heel to come off the ground throughout the movement. As the hamstring comes in the contact with the calf, the knee may cross the toe plane. If the knees are healthy, this can help to strengthen the knee as there is a greater VMO, adductor, hamstring, and gluteal activation with deeper squats and lunges. Once the back knee is 1-2" above the ground initiate the backward movement through the ball of the front foot by driving the shoulders back to the start position with no change in posture. Make sure the front heel never comes off the ground or elevated platform. Perform all reps on one leg, then perform all reps on the opposite leg.

Keys to Movement:

1. Maintain lordotic/neutral posture with torso perpendicular to floor throughout the movement.
2. Determine optimal distance between front and rear foot.
3. Focus on keeping the back leg as straight as possible to ensure maximal tension on front leg and stretching of back leg hip flexor musculature.
4. Lower down until hamstring comes in contact with calf. In healthy knees, the knee may cross of the toe plane as there is a greater recruitment of VMO, adductor, hamstring, and gluteal musculature.
5. Begin ascent by focusing on driving the shoulders/torso back and upward first.
6. Do not allow the front heel to come off during the movement.
7. Do not allow torso to lean over during the movement.

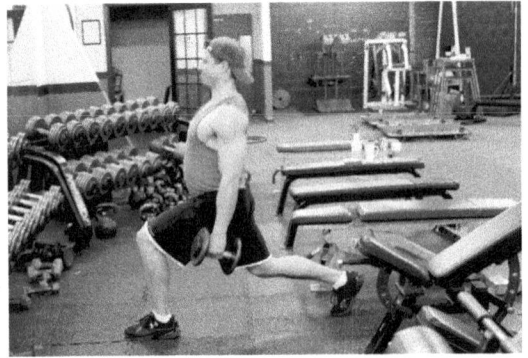

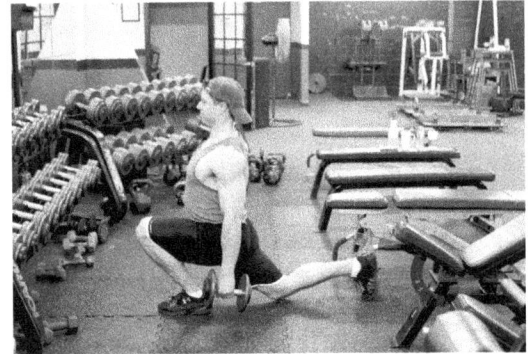

Dumbbell Squat

Classification: Lower body hip and knee extensor

Exercise Prerequisites: Glute, Hamstring, and Adductor activation. Avoid if chronic knee or low back pain.

Antagonistic Muscles to movement: Hamstrings as flexors of the knee.

Movement: Hold dumbbells by your sides with straight arms. Assume a stable neutral/lordotic posture, keeping the weight balanced between feet. Place the feet hip width apart or slightly wider, with toes pointing straight ahead or slightly out. Keep your arms straight. As you begin the descent, make sure to maintain lordotic posture beginning the decent by bending your knees first (a variation is to bend at the hips first). As you sit downward, begin pushing your knees outward to ensure maximum hip muscle recruitment. Once your hamstrings touch your calves, or you have gone as low as your flexibility allows, begin to initiate the ascent. Keeping the back arched/neutral with torso rigid, focus on driving the elbows up first, keeping the torso upright.. Be sure to keep the heels driving into the ground, and avoid caving knees and rounding of the back. Make sure to exhale maximally after you have passed the sticking point and ascend all the way to the top. Then perform next repetition.

Keys to Movement:

1. Hold dumbbells by your sides with arms straight.
2. Place feet hip width or slightly wider with toes pointing slightly outward.
3. Maintain neutral/lordotic posture while keeping the torso as upright as possible.
4. Bend at the knees first when you begin your ascent.
5. Push the knees outward, ensuring they point in the same direction as the toes throughout the movement.
6. Do not allow the heels to come off the ground or knees collapse throughout the movement.
7. Lower down until your hamstrings touch your calves or as low as your flexibility allows.

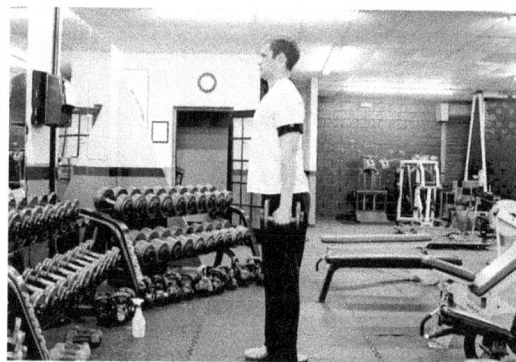

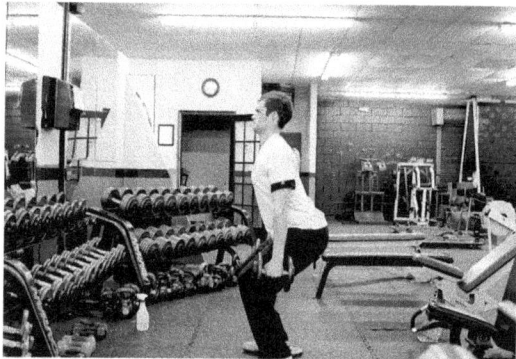

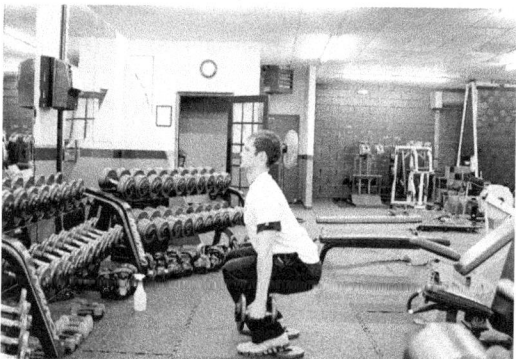

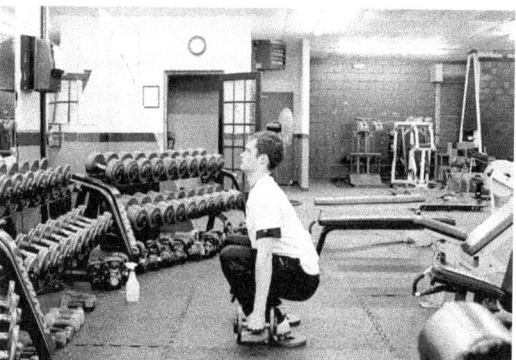

Forward Sled Dragging

Classification: Hip Extensors and Knee Extensors

Exercise Prerequisites: Avoid if you have persistent neck, knee, or low back pain.

Movement: Facing away from a sled, holding the straps by your sides with arms extended. Lean forward to about 45 degree angle relative to the floor. Feet should be feet hip width apart. Keeping the same torso position with arms straight by your sides, begin walking by driving the knee upward and landing in a modified lunge. From here focus on pulling with the hip extensors of the lead leg until the leg is straight. Drive the opposite knee high and repeat.

Keys to Movement:

1. Position feet hip width apart.
2. Lean over with torso roughly 45 degrees relative to the floor.
3. Keep arms extended by your sides.
4. Lunge step outward, driving the lead leg knee high.
5. Focus on driving forward using the lead leg hip extensor musculature.

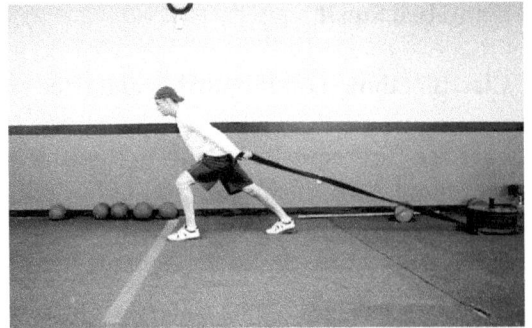

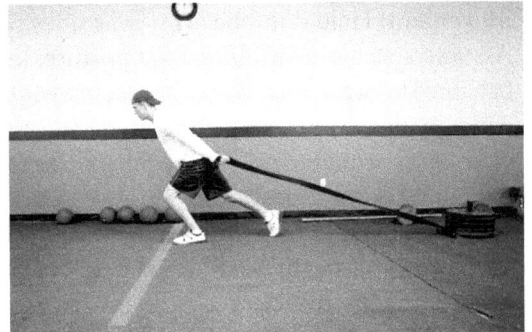

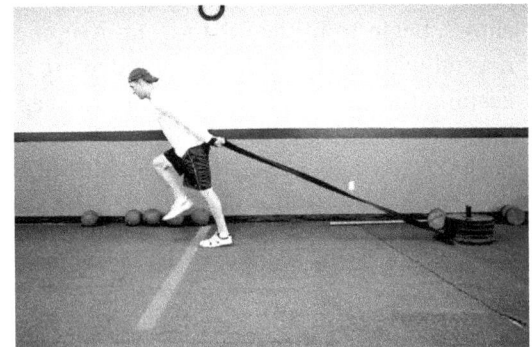

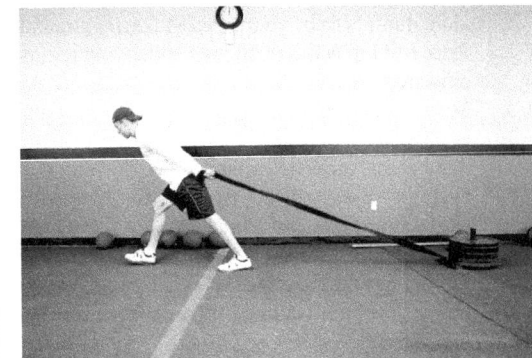

Flat Dumbbell Bench Press

Classification: Upper Body Push

Target Muscles: Pectorals, Anterior Deltoids, Triceps

Exercise Prerequisites: Avoid exercise if you experience anterior or posterior shoulder pain, or AC joint pain. If upper crossed syndrome is an issue, perform corrective movements.

Antagonistic Muscles: Rhomboids, Trap 2-4, External Rotators

Movement: The purpose of the neutral grip flat dumbbell bench press is to enhance pectoral stretch and recruitment while protecting the shoulders and enhancing triceps activation. Lie on a flat bench with feet flat on the floor. Utilizing a neutral grip with dumbbells parallel to each other and parallel to the floor, keep the angle between the upper body and upper arm to 45 degrees or less. Pinch your shoulder blades back, hugging the bench, while expanding your chest upward.

Beginning with the dumbbells in the arms extended position, begin by lowering the dumbbells straight down. Keep the dumbbells parallel to the floor and parallel to each other, while keeping the upper arm angle relative to the body at 45 degrees or less.

Lower down to your sides until the handgrips of the dumbbells are parallel to the chest. Keeping the shoulder blades pulled back, begin the concentric action, retracing the same pattern the dumbbells were lowered. Breath out on the way up, while focusing on pectoral muscle recruitment.

Do not allow the dumbbells to rotate or the elbows to flare outward during the pressing movement. Also, ensure the low back is pressed firmly against the bench to avoid neck or low back strain.

Keys to the Movement:

1. Esure dumbbells are kept parallel to each other and parallel to the floor throughout the movement.
2. Upper arm at 45 degree angle or less relative to the upper body.
3. Keep low back firmly pressed against bench.
4. Pinch shoulder blades back with chest "out" to minimize shoulder injury potential.
5. Breath out during concentric movement.

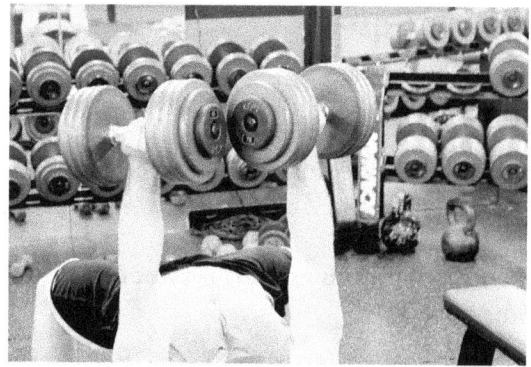

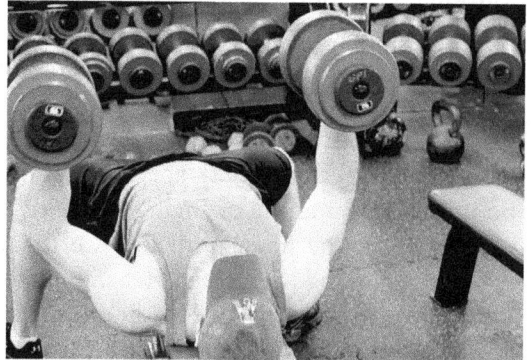

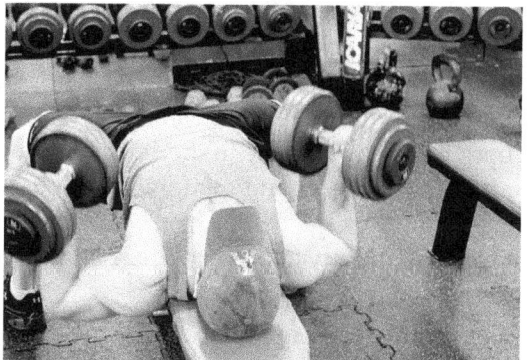

Front Squat

Classification: Lower body hip and knee extensor

Exercise Prerequisites: Glute, Hamstring, and Adductor activation. Avoid if chronic knee or low back pain.

Antagonistic Muscles to movement: Hamstrings as flexors of the knee.

Movement: Position hands in "clean" rack position, with barbell resting across upper chest and anterior deltoids. Keep upper arm parallel to the floor with elbows pointing straight forward. Once you have un-racked the bar, assume a stable neutral/lordotic posture, keeping the weight balanced between feet. Place the feet hip width apart or slightly wider, with toes pointing straight ahead or slightly out. Keep your elbows up. As you begin the descent, make sure to maintain lordotic posture beginning the decent by bending your knees first (a variation is to bend at the hips first). As you sit downward, begin pushing your knees outward to ensure maximum hip muscle recruitment. Once your hamstrings touch your calves, or you have gone as low as your flexibility allows, begin to initiate the ascent. Keeping the back arched/neutral with torso rigid, focus on driving the elbows up first, keeping the torso upright.. Be sure to keep the heels driving into the ground, and avoid caving knees and rounding of the back. Make sure to exhale maximally after you have passed the sticking point and ascend all the way to the top. Then perform next repetition.

Keys to Movement:

1. Place bar in "clean" rack position across the upper chest and anterior deltoids.
2. Place feet hip width or slightly wider with toes pointing slightly outward.
3. Keep the elbows pulled upward and pointing straight ahead.
4. Maintain neutral/lordotic posture while keeping the torso as upright as possible.
5. Bend at the knees first when you begin your ascent.
6. Push the knees outward, ensuring they point in the same direction as the toes throughout the movement.
7. Do not allow the heels to come off the ground or knees collapse throughout the movement.
8. Lower down until your hamstrings touch your calves or as low as your flexibility allows.
9. Initiate ascent by driving elbows upward.

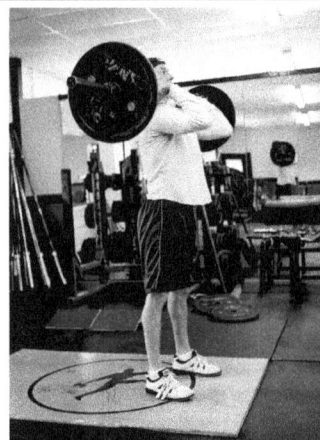

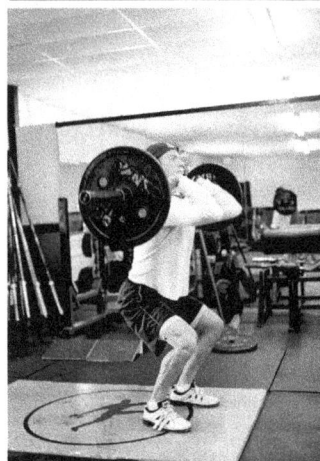

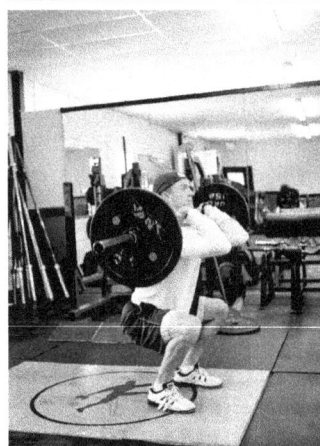

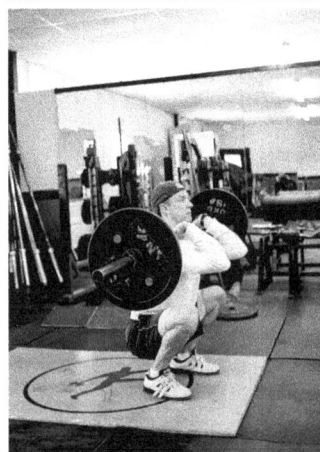

Glute Ham Raise

Classification: Posterior Chain and Hamstring as Flexor of the Knee

Exercise Prerequisites: Avoid if you have persistent knee, neck, or low back pain.

Movement: Lie on a glute ham raise machine with heels locked into pads, feet against foot plate, and quads across support pad. Lock your torso tight, maintaining neutral/slightly lordotic posture throughout. With legs extended, lower your torso downward by flexing at the hips only. From here, contact your glutes, keep your torso rigid, and begin hip extension upward. Do not shoot butt backward by bending at the hips. After your hips have reached full or near-full extension, begin flexing the knees, similar to a hamstring curl. Curl your extended torso upward until you are perpendicular to the floor. Lower back to start.

Keys to Movement:

1. Keep neutral/slightly lordotic posture throughout movement.
2. Extend legs at the bottom end range of the movement.
3. Do not bend at the hips when pulling yourself upward.
4. Contract the glutes for greater stability and hamstring activation.
5. Pull with your hamstrings until you are perpendicular to the floor.

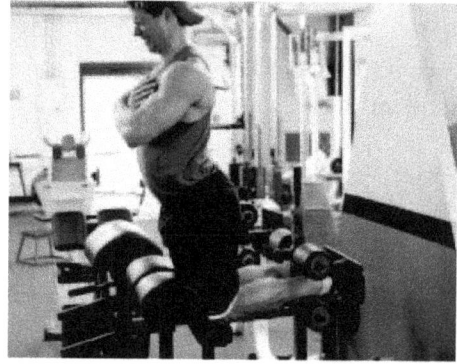

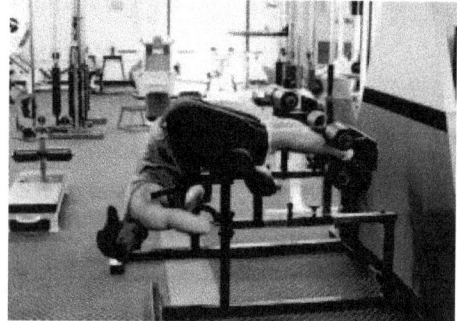

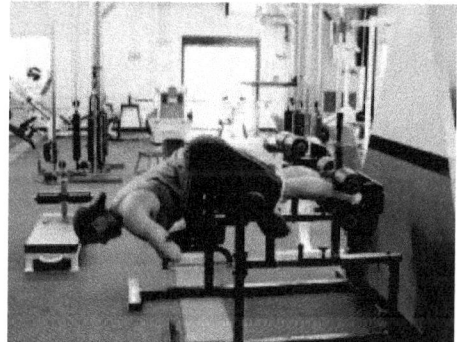

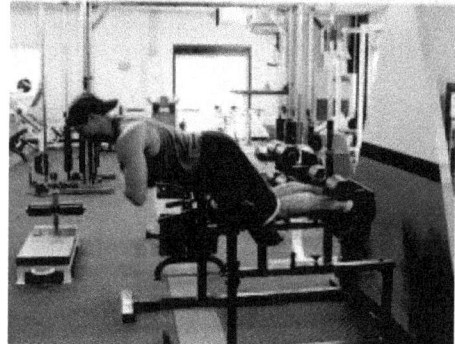

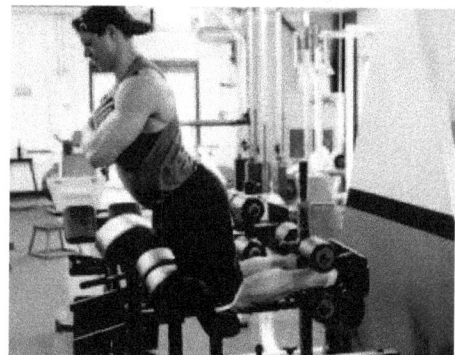

Hamstring Curls

Classification: Posterior Chain and knee flexor

Exercise Prerequisites: Avoid if you have persistent neck, knee, or low back pain.

Antagonistic Muscles to movement: Knee Extensors, Hip Flexors

Movement: Hamstring curl options include:
- Prone hamstring curl machine
- Seated hamstring curl machine
- Kneeling hamstring curl machine
- Standing hamstring curl machine

Each of these machines isolates the hamstrings in a slightly different manner. For those with structural imbalances about the hamstrings, unilateral training may be the best option for correcting these imbalances. For each hamstring curl option, control of the torso, femur position, and foot placement are critical. During any of these, do not allow the torso to generate momentum by swinging. Maintain a rigid position throughout. Also, do not allow the hamstring to generate momentum by extending the femur backward (hip extension) during the movement. Maintain the same femur position relative to the torso throughout the movement.

Adjusting the direction the toes point during hamstring curls can aid in correcting structural imbalances throughout the hamstrings. Feet inverted, everted, or neutral are the options. Also, plantar flexing the ankle can aid in minimizing gastroc recruitment throughout the movement.

Keys to Movement:

1. Rigid torso position throughout the movement. Do not allow the torso to swing or generate momentum.
2. Femur position is locked. Do not allow to swing backward to generate momentum.
3. Structural imbalances can be corrected by altering the direction the toes are pointing.
4. Plantar flexion can aid in minimizing gastroc recruitment.

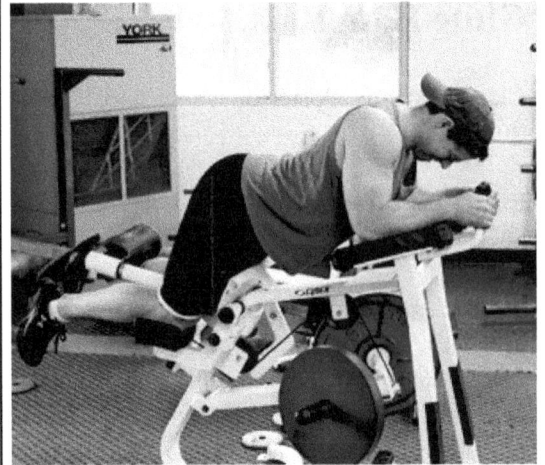

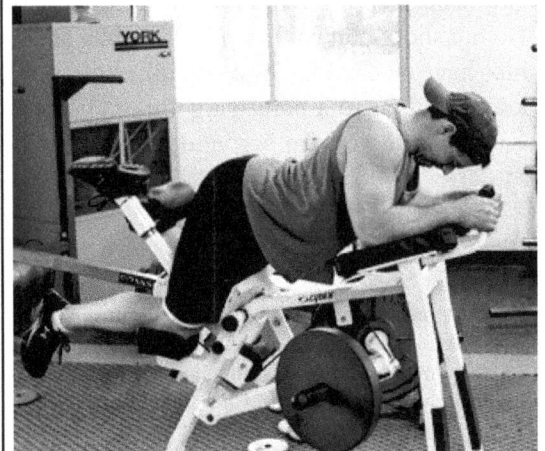

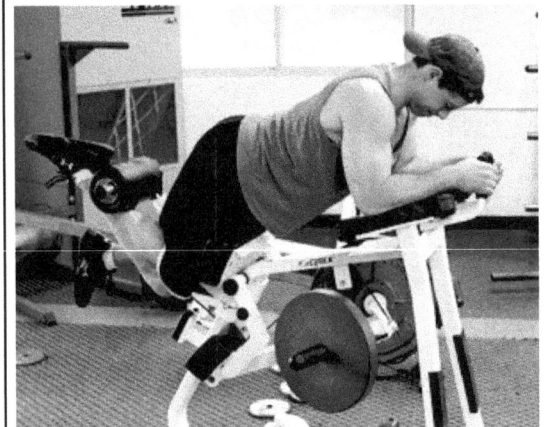

Heels Elevated Dumbbell Squat

Classification: Lower body hip and knee extensor

Exercise Prerequisites: Glute, Hamstring, and Adductor activation. Avoid if chronic knee or low back pain.

Antagonistic Muscles to movement: Hamstrings as flexors of the knee.

Movement: Hold dumbbells by your sides with straight arms. Stand with heels elevated on a ramp or weight plate. Assume a stable neutral/lordotic posture, keeping the weight balanced between feet. Place the feet hip width apart or slightly wider, with toes pointing straight ahead or slightly out. Keep your arms straight. As you begin the descent, make sure to maintain lordotic posture beginning the decent by bending your knees first (a variation is to bend at the hips first). As you sit downward, begin pushing your knees outward to ensure maximum hip muscle recruitment. Once your hamstrings touch your calves, or you have gone as low as your flexibility allows, begin to initiate the ascent. Keeping the back arched/neutral with torso rigid, focus on driving the elbows up first, keeping the torso upright.. Be sure to keep the heels driving into the ground, and avoid caving knees and rounding of the back. Make sure to exhale maximally after you have passed the sticking point and ascend all the way to the top. Then perform next repetition.

Keys to Movement:

1. Hold dumbbells by your sides with arms straight.
2. Place feet hip width or slightly wider with toes pointing slightly outward.
3. Maintain neutral/lordotic posture while keeping the torso as upright as possible.
4. Bend at the knees first when you begin your ascent.
5. Push the knees outward, ensuring they point in the same direction as the toes throughout the movement.
6. Do not allow the heels to come off the ground or knees collapse throughout the movement.
7. Lower down until your hamstrings touch your calves or as low as your flexibility allows.

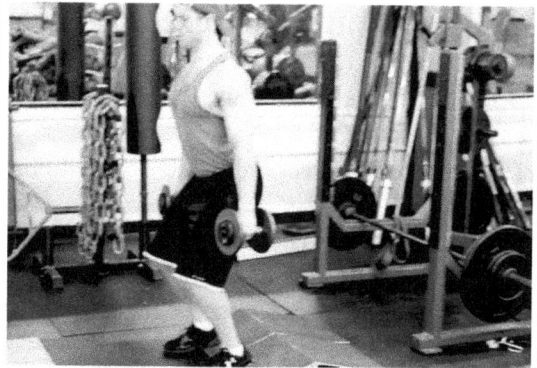

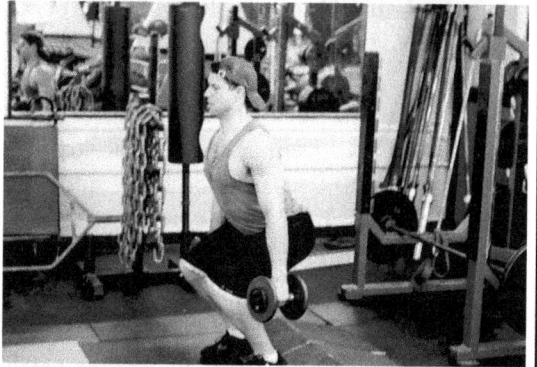

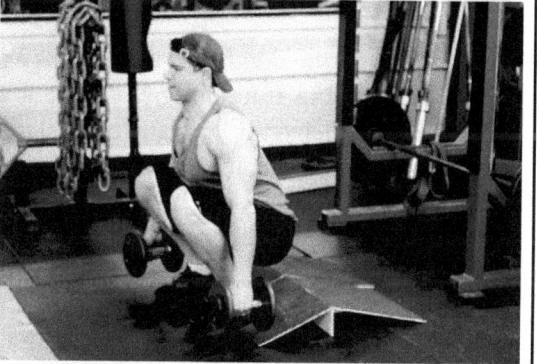

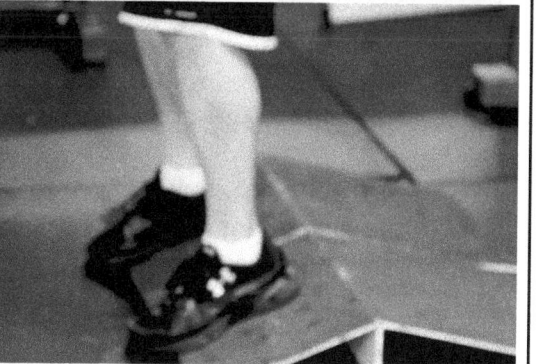

Incline Dumbbell Bench Press

Classification: Upper Body Push

Target Muscles: Pectorals, Anterior Deltoids, Triceps

Exercise Prerequisites: Avoid exercise if you experience anterior or posterior shoulder pain, or AC joint pain. If upper crossed syndrome is an issue, perform corrective movements.

Antagonistic Muscles: Rhomboids, Trap 2-4, External Rotators

Movement: The purpose of the neutral grip Incline dumbbell bench press is to enhance pectoral stretch and recruitment while protecting the shoulders and enhancing triceps activation. Lie on an incline bench with feet flat on the floor. Utilizing a neutral grip with dumbbells parallel to each other and parallel to the floor, keep the angle between the upper body and upper arm to 45 degrees or less. Pinch your shoulder blades back, hugging the bench, while expanding your chest upward.

Beginning with the dumbbells in the arms extended position, begin by lowering the dumbbells straight down. Keep the dumbbells parallel to the floor and parallel to each other, while keeping the upper arm angle relative to the body at 45 degrees or less.

Lower down to your sides until the handgrips of the dumbbells are parallel to the chest. Keeping the shoulder blades pulled back, begin the concentric action, retracing the same pattern the dumbbells were lowered. Breath out on the way up, while focusing on pectoral muscle recruitment.

Do not allow the dumbbells to rotate or the elbows to flare outward during the pressing movement. Also, ensure the low back is pressed firmly against the bench to avoid neck or low back strain.

Keys to the Movement
1. Ensure dumbbells are kept parallel to each other and parallel to the floor throughout the movement.
2. Upper arm at 45 degree angle or less relative to the upper body.
3. Keep low back firmly pressed against bench.
4. Pinch shoulder blades back with chest "out" to minimize shoulder injury potential.
5. Breath out during concentric movement.

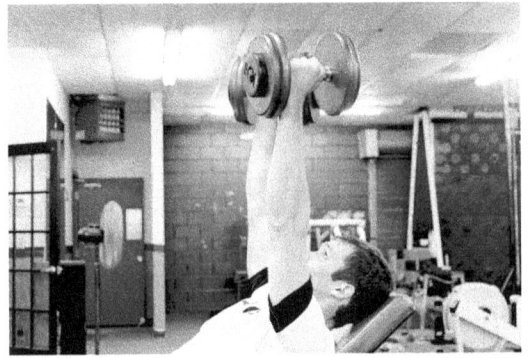

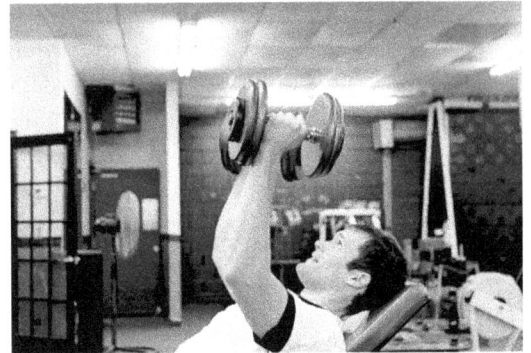

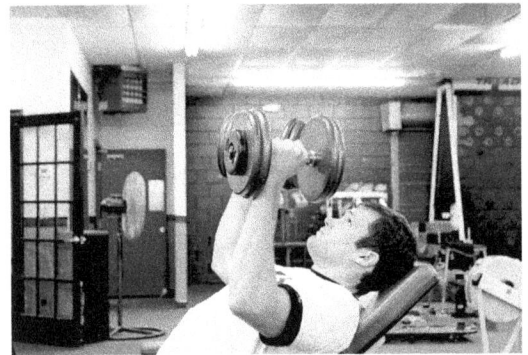

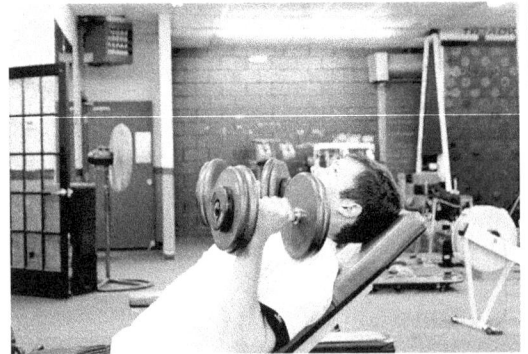

Inverted Row

Classification: Upper Posterior Chain Pull Movement

Target Muscles: Trapezius, Latissimus Dorsi, Rhomboids, Rear Delts, Posterior Rotator Cuff Muscles, Low Back Extensor Chain

Exercise Prerequisites: Correct activation of glutes, hamstrings, low back extensors, rear deltoids, lats, and rhomboids. Avoid if you have persistent, low back, elbow, or shoulder pain

Antagonistic Muscles to movement: Shoulder internal rotators and elbow extensors.

Movement: Position fixed Olympic bar 2-3 feet off the ground. Lay on your back with your (heels) resting on the floor or on a Swiss ball. With pronated grip, grasp the bar slightly wider than shoulder width. Extend hips and push chest out so body is in neutral/slightly lordotic posture. Maintaining posture, pull chest to bar, initiating movement by retracting the shoulder blades and driving the elbows back. Once your chest makes contact with the bar, slowly lower back to start without breaking posture.

Movement Mechanics:

1. Grasp bar with pronated grip and hands slightly wider than shoulder width.
2. Extend hips and keep back in lordotic/neutral posture.
3. Do not allow hips to flex throughout movement.
4. Retract shoulder blades and pull chest to the bar.
5. Lower back to start position.

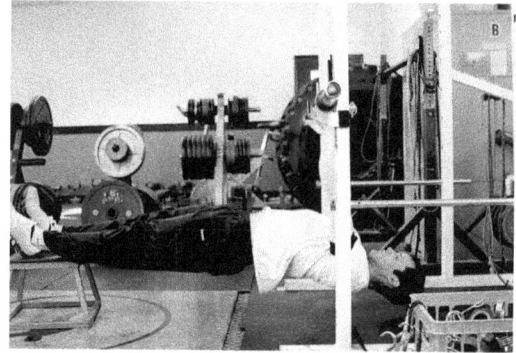

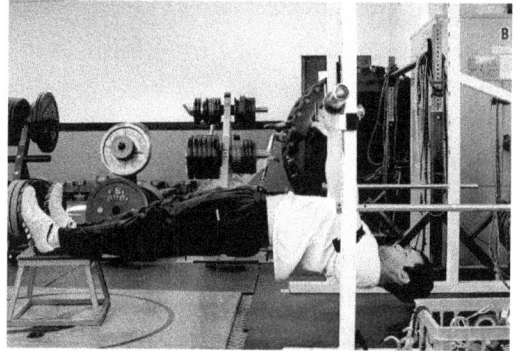

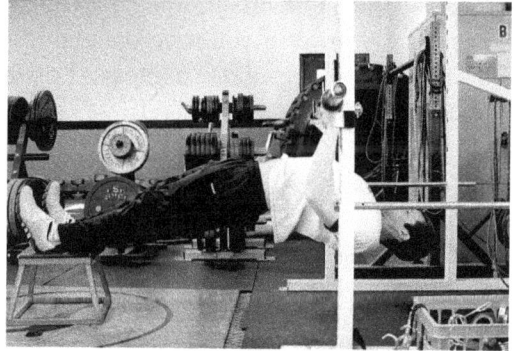

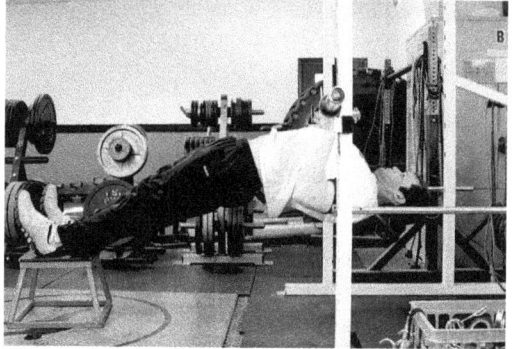

Leg Press

Classification: Bilateral Posterior Chain and knee Extensor

Exercise Prerequisites: Avoid if you have persistent neck, knee, or low back pain

Antagonistic Muscles to movement: Hamstrings as flexors of the knee.

Movement: Lay back on a 45 degree leg press machine. Position feet hip width apart with majority of the weight on the back half of the foot. Do not allow the butt come off the back of the pad. Initiate the movement from the glutes and hamstrings by driving through the heels first. Keeping your head back, low back pushed firmly against the back of the machine, extend the legs to 160 to 170 degree angle at the knees. You do not want to fully extend or hyperextend as the weight may be too much for your knee joints to handle and could cause injury. Lower down to the point where the upper thigh is parallel or just below parallel to the foot plate. You may also go lower if you have optimal hip mobility and the low back does not round or come off the bench. Repeat for the required repetitions.

Keys to Movement:

1. Press low back firmly against pad.
2. Ensure that knees are pointing in the same direction as the toes throughout the movement.
3. Keep the heels in contact with the plate.
4. Lower to the point where the upper thigh is parallel to the plate or as low as your hips allow you to travel without low back rounding or coming off the pad.

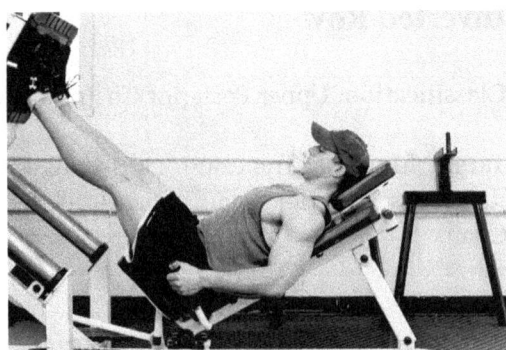

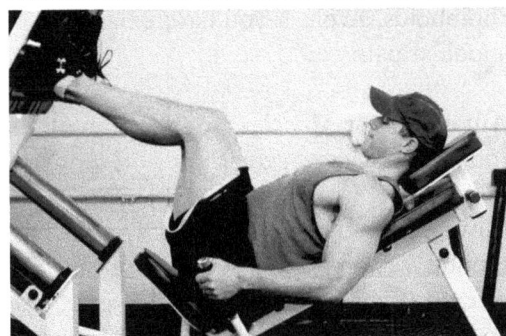

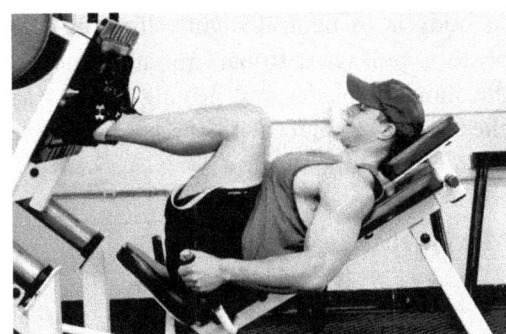

Low Back Extension

Classification: Posterior Chain and knee Extensor

Exercise Prerequisites: Avoid if you have persistent neck, knee, or low back pain.

Antagonistic Muscles to movement: Hamstrings as flexors of the knee.

Movement: Position yourself on a conventional hyperextension machine or a 45 degree back extension machine. Make sure the thighs are prone on the pad with the calves or Achilles tendons under the brace pads. Holding a lordotic/neutral spine, lower your body straight down until reaching roughly 90 degree hip flexion or until you cannot hold lordotic posture. Initiate the concentric movement by contracting the glutes and hamstrings while maintaining lordotic/neutral posture. Only raise until your torso reaches neutral position. Do not hyperextend.

Keys to Movement:

1. Hold lordotic/neutral posture throughout movement.
2. Lower down until you can no longer hold lordotic/neutral posture.
3. Initiate concentric movement by engaging the glutes and hamstrings first.
4. Raise up until you reach neutral starting position. Do not hyperextend.

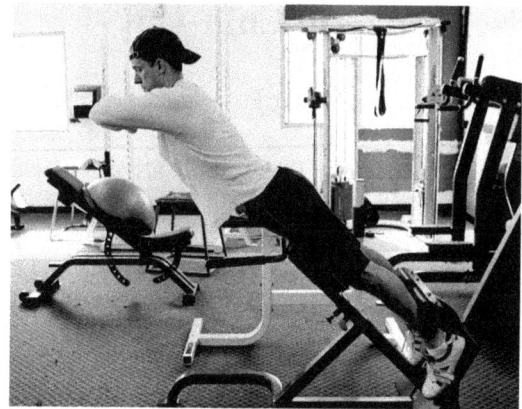

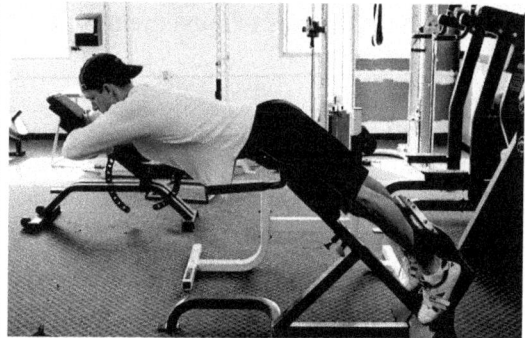

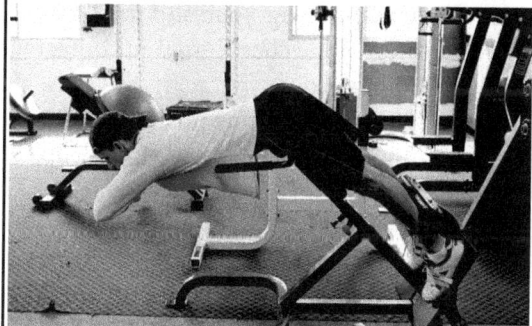

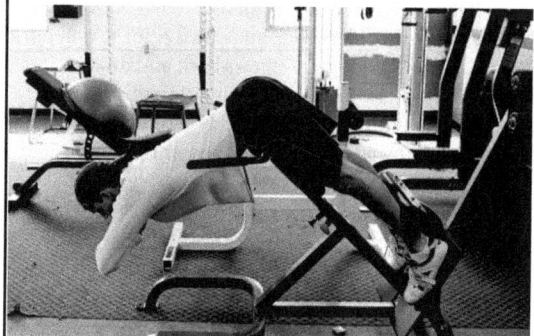

Neutral Grip Chin-Ups

Classification: Upper Posterior Chain Pull Movement

Target Muscles: Trapezius, Latissimus Dorsi, Rhomboids, Levator Scapulae, Brachialis, Biceps Brachii

Exercise Prerequisites: Correct activation of Latissimus Dorsi and rhomboids. Do not do if you have elbow, shoulder or serious low back pain

Antagonistic Muscles to movement: Internal rotators, elbow extensors

Movement: Grasp a neutral grip pull-up bar with hands neutral, shoulder width or slightly wider. Hang from the bar, with arms, hips and shoulders in complete extension. Initiate movement by retracting shoulder blades back and down. Begin pulling your body straight upward, continuing to pull the shoulder blades back and downward. Do not allow the shoulder to internally rotate as you are pulling upward.
Pull upward, pinching your shoulder blades back until the upper portion of the chest comes in contact with the bar.
Lower the body slowly, retracing the same pattern until you reach full extension starting position at the bottom.
If you cannot perform a regular chin-up, you can use the assistance of a partner or a band around the knee or foot.

Movement Mechanics:

1. Neutral grip with hands shoulder width or slightly closer.
2. Begin in "dead hang" position.
3. Retract shoulders back and down prior to and during the movement.
4. Focus on pulling the elbows back and down.
5. Do not allow the shoulders to internally rotate,
6. Pull up until upper part of chest comes in contact with the bar.
7. Lower down until full extension in the elbows and shoulders.

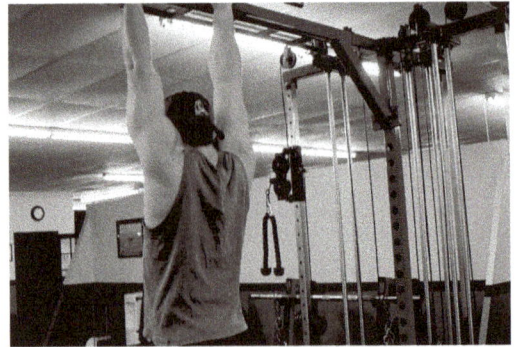

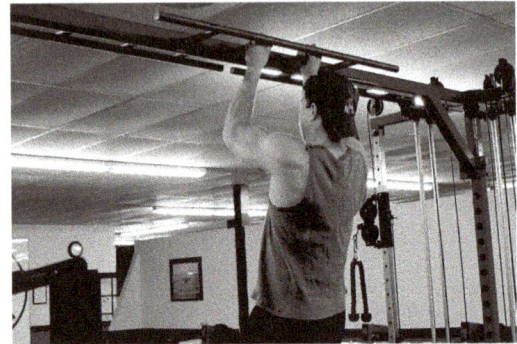

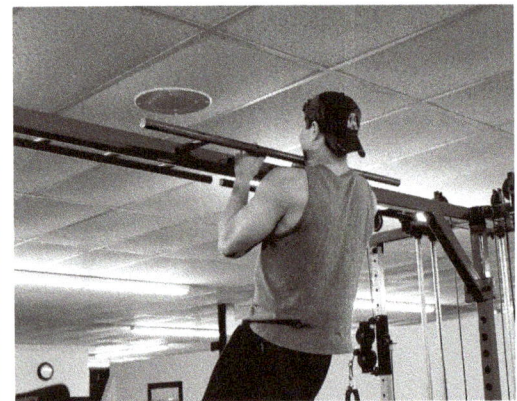

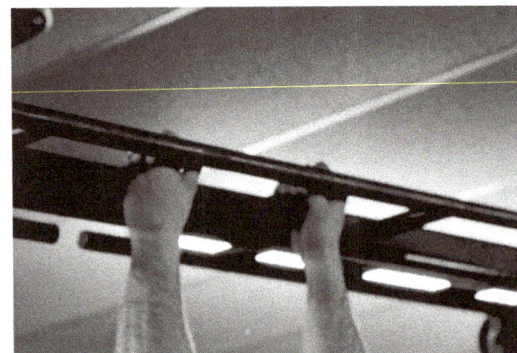

Off Bench Oblique

Classification: Low Back, Core, and oblique

Exercise Prerequisites: Avoid if you have persistent knee, shoulder, neck, or low back pain.

Movement: More than just an oblique exercise, this exercise strengthens the powerful Quadratus Lumborum muscles of the low back. When strong, these muscles provide the soccer athlete with the upright stability necessary for maintaining possession or knocking the opponent off the ball. Lay down on your side on a bench, with the upper body hanging off the bench and heels/legs anchored under an immovable bar. Fold your arms across your chest or position your hands at your ears and lower your torso/shoulder toward the ground keeping your shoulders/torso perpendicular to floor and parallel to the walls. Once the eccentric component is complete, pull our torso up as high as you can, maintaining the same perpendicular to the floor and parallel to the wall posture. Variations to this exercise include feet stacked on top of each other, one foot in front of the other, isometric hold at the top of concentric contraction, or holding a weight in your arms across the chest.

Keys to Movement:

1. Lie on your side with feet anchored either stacked, bottom leg in front, or bottom leg in back.
2. Keep hips squared to wall and perpendicular to the floor. Do not allow your hips to rotate forward or backward.
3. Fold arms across your chest.
4. Keeping torso parallel to a wall, lower your shoulder closest to the floor downward.
5. Once you have reached full stretch, pull your torso upward, pulling slightly past neutral posture.

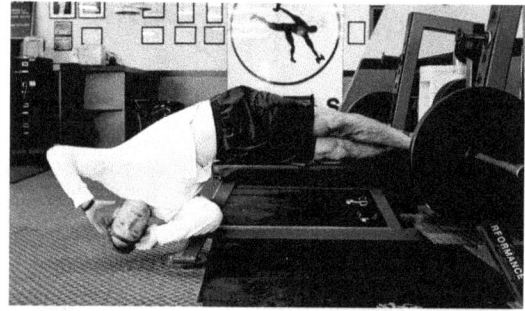

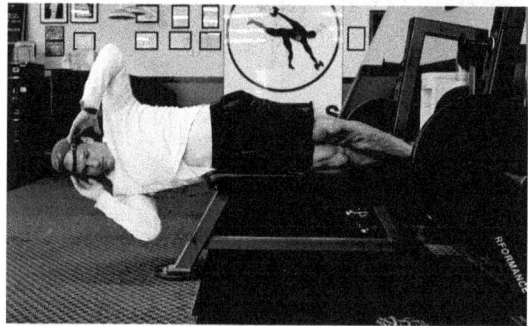

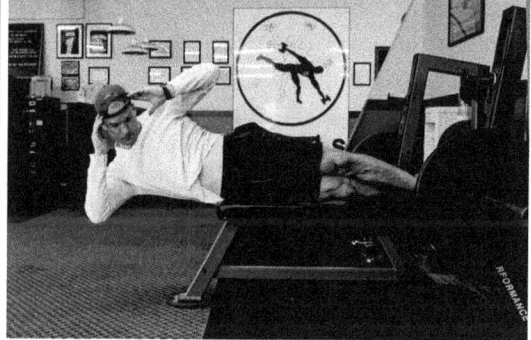

One Arm Dumbbell Row

Classification: Upper Posterior Chain Pull Movement

Target Muscles: Trapezius, Latissimus Dorsi, Rhomboids, Rear Delts, Posterior Rotator Cuff Muscles, Low Back Extensor Chain

Exercise Prerequisites: Correct activation of rear deltoids, rhomboids, and latissimus musculature. Avoid movement if you have low back pain

Antagonistic Muscles to movement: Shoulder internal rotators, elbow extensors.

Movement: Lean torso over until parallel or less than 45 degree angle relative to the floor. Stagger feet with foot on side of the hand holding the dumbbell in back. Brace opposite arm against a stable object to aid in holding the torso in position. Hold a dumbbell with neutral grip, knees bent roughly 20 degrees. Arch your back into a lordotic posture, with chest out, shoulder pulled back and down, eyes straight down.
Maintaining torso position relative to the floor with lordotic posture, pull the weight to your side toward your sternum/ belly button, activating first the rear delt muscles, then pulling with the larger rhomboid and lat muscles. To do this, retract your shoulder blades back and down, then focus on pulling back with the elbows until full contraction of the upper back musculature.
Ensure not to allow the shoulders to shrug upward as this takes away from the contraction of the mid back/shoulder retractor muscles. Make sure there is no bounce or rounding of the back throughout the movement. Slowly lower the weight back to the start position and perform next repetition.

Keys to Movement:

1. Position body in correct starting position with knees bent 20 degrees, chest out, back arched, torso parallel or near parallel to the floor, and feet staggered.
2. Initiate movement by retracting shoulders back and down, maintaining torso posture.
3. Focus on pulling elbows back.
4. Do not allow shoulders to shrug upward.
5. Row back until complete contraction of shoulder blades.

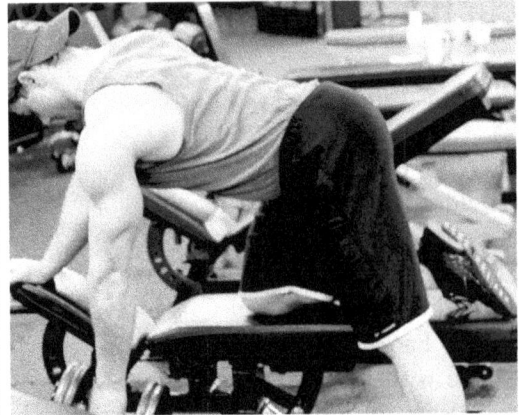

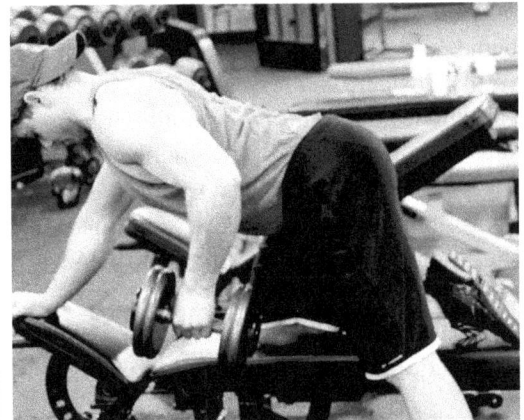

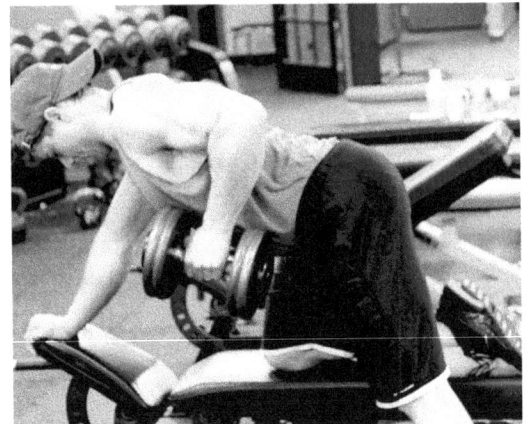

Palloff Press

Classification: Anti Torso Rotation

Exercise Prerequisites: Avoid if you have persistent shoulder, neck, or low back pain.

Movement: Adjust a cable column to sternum height. Stand sideways roughly three feet from the column. Grasp D handle with arm/hand furthest from the column on first. Hand on adjacent side is placed on top of opposite hand. Position your feet hip width or slightly wider with knees slightly bent. Keeping torso rigid and locked upright, start with your fists at your sternum. Begin pressing straight outward. Do not allow the resistance from the cable to rotate your torso or pull your arms toward the column. Fully extend your arms and return to start.

Keys to Movement:

1. Stand sideways roughly 3 feet from a cable column.
2. Opposite hand grasps the D handle first. Adjacent hand is on top.
3. Position feet hip width or slightly wider.
4. Lock torso, square hips, and bend knees slightly.
5. Press straight outward from sternum height.
6. Do not allow the torso to rotate or arms to be pulled toward the cable column.

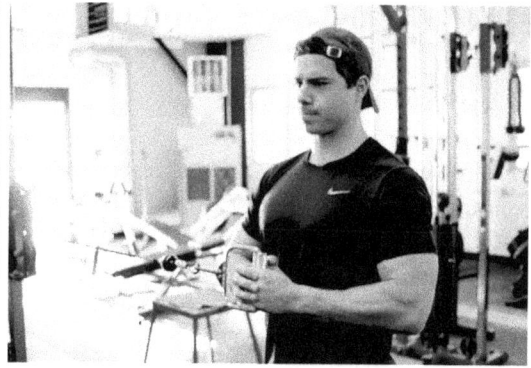

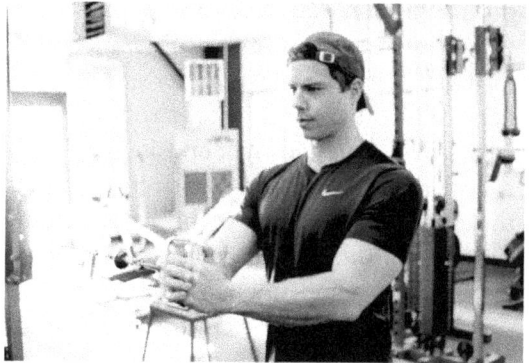

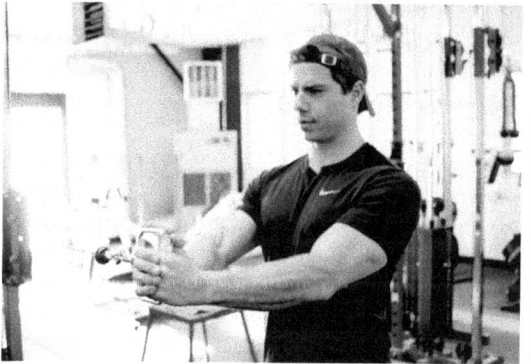

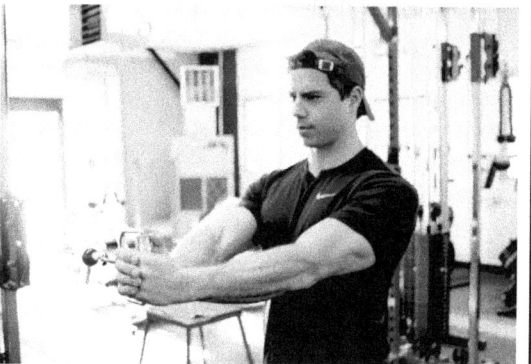

PNF Chop

Classification: Rotational

Exercise Prerequisites: Avoid if you have persistent knee, shoulder, neck, or low back pain.

Movement: Adjust a cable column to a high position. Attach a triceps rope. Offset the rope with the cable attachment ring at the top of the rope with the rest of the rope hanging down. Position your body into a hip flexor stretch position, with your leg opposite the column behind and adjacent leg forward. Keeping your torso upright, grasp the rope with your hand adjacent at the top of the rope directly next to the cable attachment ring and the opposite hand at the bottom of the rope. Keeping your hip flexor stretched and torso upright, pull the cable to your chest with both arms. Your hand adjacent to the column should end up at your sternum while your hand opposite is out and down to your side.

From here press downward to your side until your adjacent hand is parallel to your opposite hip. The other hand should be slightly behind you at glute height. Return to start.

Keys to Movement:

1. Position your body sideways to a cable column in a hip flexor stretch position with opposite leg back and adjacent leg forward.
2. Keeping torso upright, pull cable across body until adjacent hand is at your sternum and opposite hand at your side.
3. Press downward until adjacent hand his parallel to adjacent hip. The other hand should be behind your glutes.
4. Ensure that you are stretching your hip flexor and keeping torso upright throughout the movement.

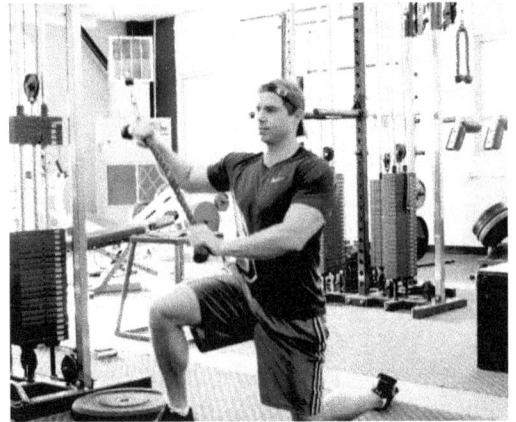

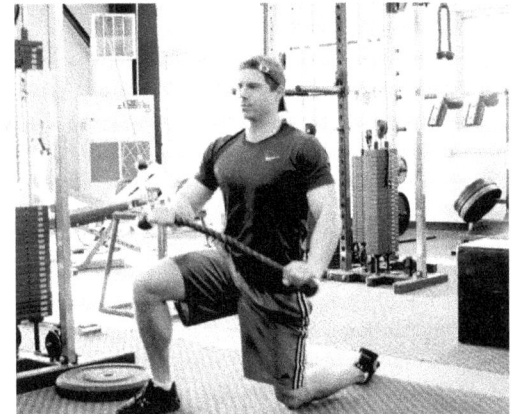

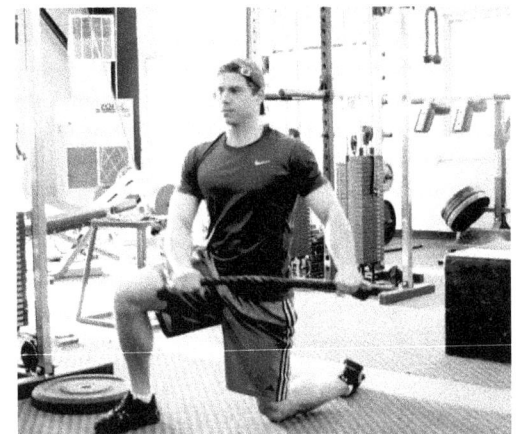

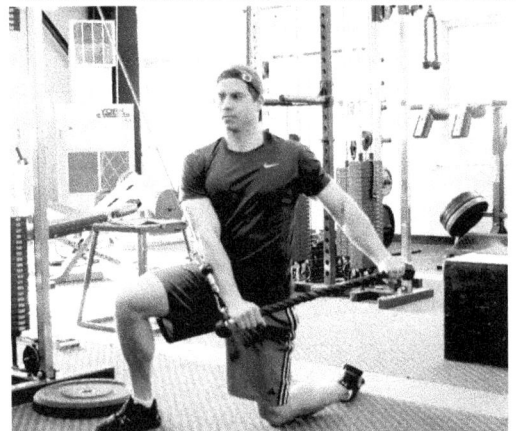

PNF Rotational Lift

Classification: Rotational

Exercise Prerequisites: Avoid if you have persistent knee, shoulder, neck, or low back pain.

Movement: Adjust a cable column to the bottom position. Attach a D handle. Stand sideways next to the column with feet roughly hip width apart. Grasp the D handle with the opposite hand on first and adjacent hand on top with arms extended. With a slight bend in the knee and torso in rigid upright position, begin pulling the cable in a rotational direction upward, initiating the pull through the ground reaction forces against the ball of the foot on the foot closest to the cable column. Pivot the back foot and rotate the hips until your hips and shoulders are parallel to the column with arms extended outward overhead. The movement is slightly similar to that of a golf swing in which the hips and shoulders rotate.

Keys to Movement:

1. Stand sideways next to a cable column with feet hip width apart.
2. Grasp the D handle with the opposite hand first and adjacent hand on top.
3. Initiate the movement by driving through the ball of the back foot.
4. Bring the cable in a circular fashion similar to that of a golf swing.
5. Rotate the hips and shoulders until they are parallel to the column.
6. Finish with the arms extended outward and upward over your head with hips and shoulders squared to the cable column.

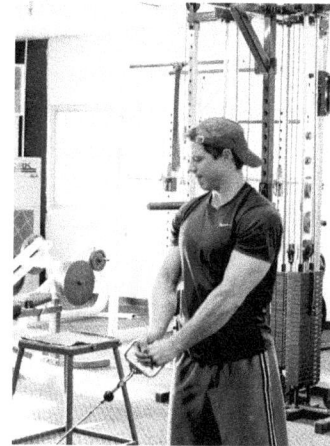

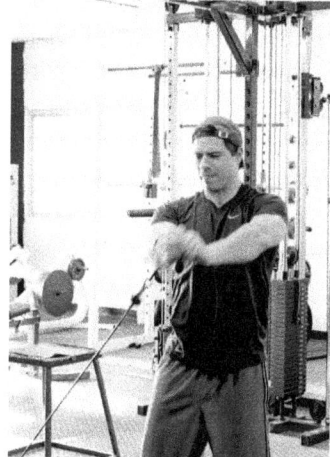

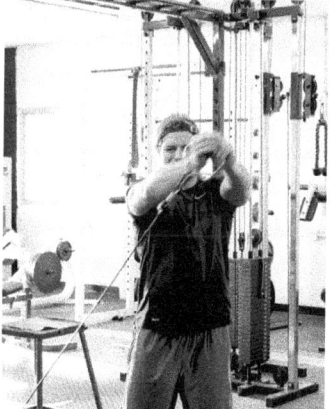

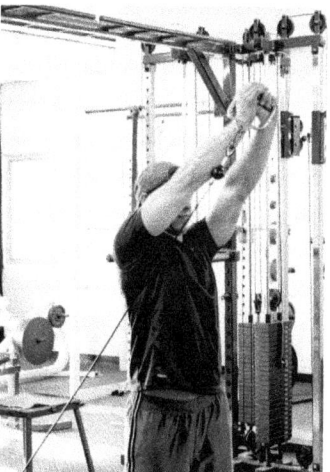

Peterson Step Ups

Classification: Knee Extensors

Exercise Prerequisites: Avoid if you have persistent knee or low back pain

Antagonistic Muscles to movement: Hamstrings as flexors of the knee.

Movement: Stand on a 2-5 inch platform, with other foot on the floor. Lift the heel of the foot on the platform as high as you can, distributing the weight through the toes and ball of the foot. Extend your hips completely, maintaining a straight line from knee to hip to shoulder on the leg on the plafrorm. Extend the knee of the elevated leg, rasing the other foot off the ground. Try to keep your heel elevated as long as possible on the elevated leg. Drop the heel to the platform once the feet are even. Lower back to start. Focus on keeping the hips extended to avoid excessive torque

Keys to Movement:

1. Keep weight on the ball of the foot to ensure recruitment of the VMO
2. Knee points in same direction as the toes throughout the movement..
3. Keep hips extended throughout the movement.
4. Do not use the other foot for assistance.

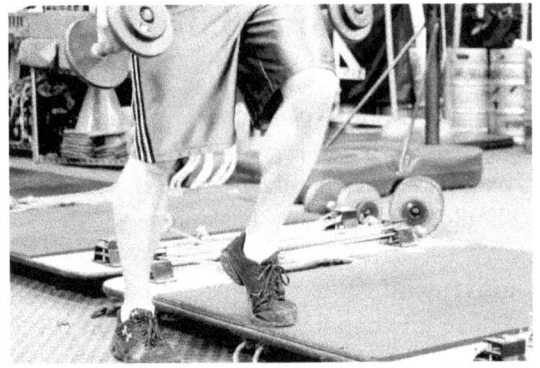

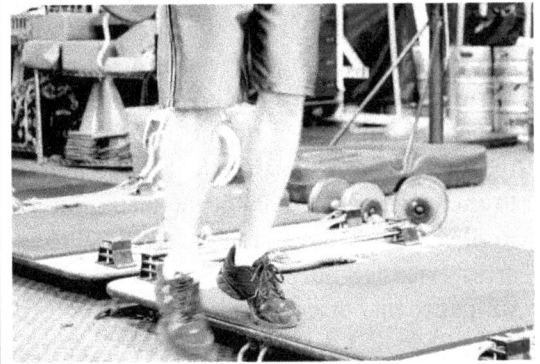

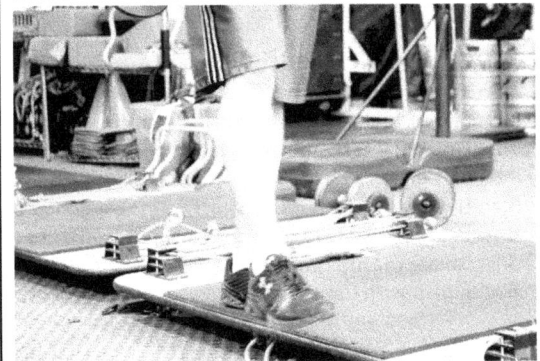

Power Clean/Full Clean from the Hang

Classification: Total Body Power

Exercise Prerequisites: Avoid if you have persistent neck, knee, or low back pain.

Movement:
Start Position:
Feet shoulder width apart with toes pointed slightly out. Feet should be flat on the ground, with pressure toward the balls of the feet.

Back should be arched or flat with bar directly over the instep of your foot.

Hips should be higher than the knees

Shoulders and knees should be out over or past the bar.

Hands are wide with hook grip, elbows turned out and wrists slightly flexed.

Head should be neutral, focusing on a point straight ahead.

1st Pull
* Maintaining neutral or arched back, the bar is raised by extending the knees, allowing the knees to come behind the bar.
* The shoulders remain over the bar, with elbows turned out and wrists remaining slightly flexed.

2nd Knee Bend
* This occurs between knee and mid thigh, with a re-bending of the knees (this is the second knee bend of the double knee bend) creating a mild "unloading" effect.
* The body is basically re-aligned to position itself for greater vertical force production.
* The bar is then pulled to mid thigh.

2nd Pull
* The hips are powerfully extended
* The feet are plantar flexed pushing the toes and balls of the feet into the ground.
* The shoulders are shrugged toward the ears
* Elbows are still rotated outward with wrists trying to hold flexed position.

The Catch
* The body drops under the bar into an overhead squat maintaining a neutral/lordotic posture
* Arms are straight, with the bar overhead.
* Hands, elbows, and shoulders are externally rotated
* Heel foot strike to ensure feet land flat on the ground.
* Eyes looking straight ahead with head neutral.

Variations:
1. "Hang" refers to variations in start ranging from below the knee, above the knee, mid thigh, etc..
2. Power Snatch refers to a catch that does not result in deep overhead squat, with the tops of the thighs above parallel. This exercise is more common in training and testing for sport as it reflects powerful pulling/triple extension rather than flexibility and front squat strength.
3. "From the blocks" refers to a start position directly off a measured box height.

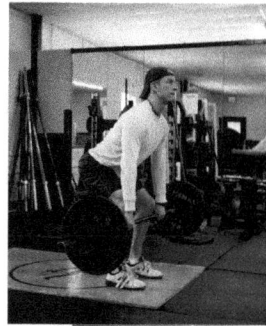

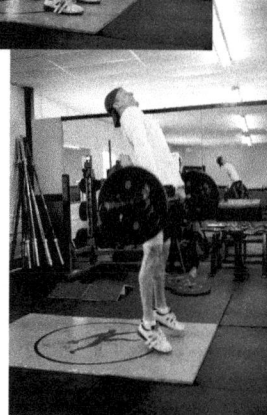

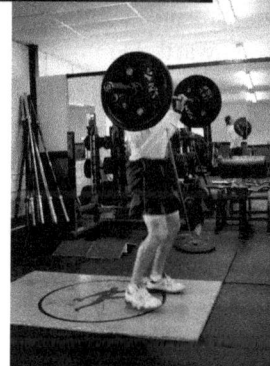

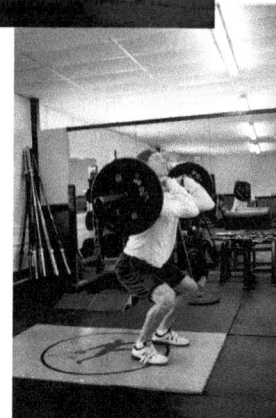

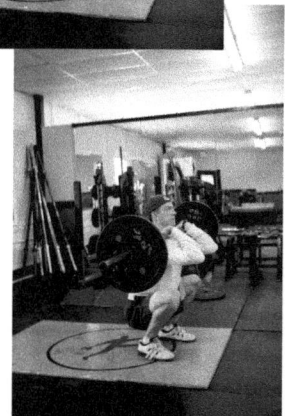

Pull-ups

Classification: Upper Posterior Chain Pull Movement

Target Muscles: Trapezius, Latissimus Dorsi, Rhomboids, Levator Scapulae, Brachialis, Biceps Brachii

Exercise Prerequisites: Correct activation of Latissimus Dorsi and rhomboids. Do not do if you have elbow, shoulder or serious low back pain

Antagonistic Muscles to movement: Internal rotators, elbow extensors

Movement: Grasp a pull-up bar with hands pronated, shoulder width or slightly wider. Hang from the bar, with arms, hips and shoulders in complete extension. Initiate movement by retracting shoulder blades back and down. Begin pulling your body straight upward, continuing to pull the shoulder blades back and downward. Do not allow the shoulder to internally rotate as you are pulling upward.

Pull upward, pinching your shoulder blades back until the upper portion of the chest comes in contact with the bar.

Lower the body slowly, retracing the same pattern until you reach full extension starting position at the bottom.

If you cannot perform a regular pull-up, you can use the assistance of a partner or a band around the knee or foot.

Keys to Movement:

1. Pronated grip with hands shoulder width or slightly wider.
2. Begin in "dead hang" position.
3. Retract shoulders back and down prior to and during the movement.
4. Focus on pulling the elbows back and down.
5. Do not allow the shoulders to internally rotate,
6. Pull up until upper part of chest comes in contact with the bar.
7. Lower down until full extension in the elbows and shoulders.

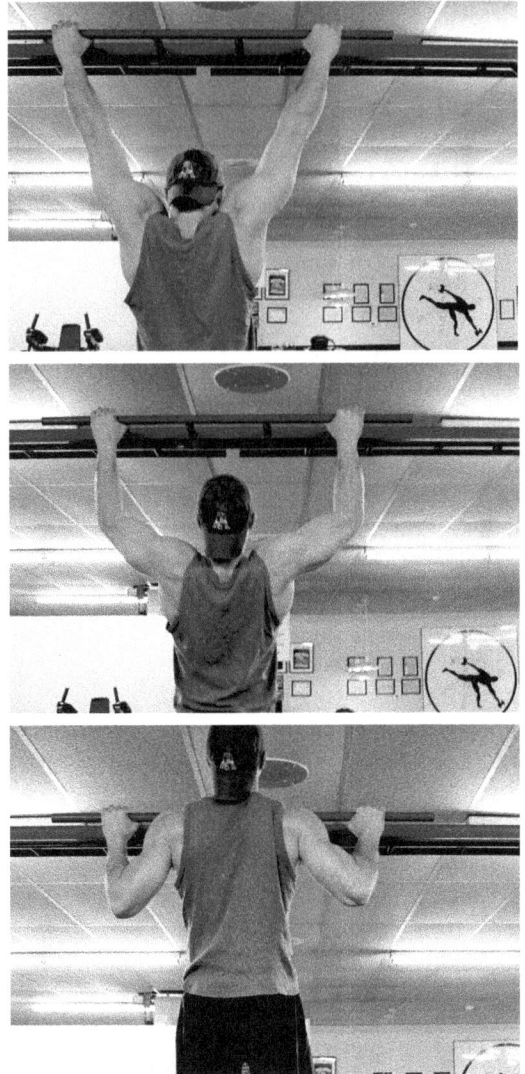

Push Jerk (or split jerk)

Classification: Upper Body Press

Exercise Prerequisites: Avoid if you have persistent neck, knee, or low back pain.

Movement: Stand with feet in hip width staggered stance or hip width parallel stance. Hold barbell with pronated grip (palms forward). Begin with your upper arms pointing downward/slightly forward with triceps making contact with lats. The barbell should rest on the front anterior deltoid and upper chest musculature. Keeping the pelvis neutral, heels in contact with the floor, torso rigid, and eyes straight, explosively bend knees 10-20 degrees. Immediately reverse direction, driving through the legs and hips to generate momentum. Carry the momentum generated through the legs and hips and press the bar straight upward. At the same time you are pressing the bar upward, push the body under the bar by re-bending the knees. Once the barbell has passed the top of your head, tuck your chin downward, gazing down at the ground roughly 5-10 feet in front of you (make sure not to hit your head with the bar). Continue pressing straight upward, until you have reached full extension of the arms and shoulders. Try to bring your shoulders to ear height at the top of the movement. Once you reach top position, you should catch the bar in a knees bent position. Slowly lower back to start.

Keys to Movement:

1. Keep torso upright throughout entire movement.
2. Hold barbell in pronated grip.
3. Triceps in contact with lats at the beginning of the movement.
4. Quick knee bend, followed by extension to generate momentum from the legs and hips.
5. Tuck your chin once the barbell has passed the top of your head.
6. Do not allow your back to arch as you press overhead.
7. "Active" shoulders at the top.
8. Push yourself under the bar, catching the bar in a knees bent position.

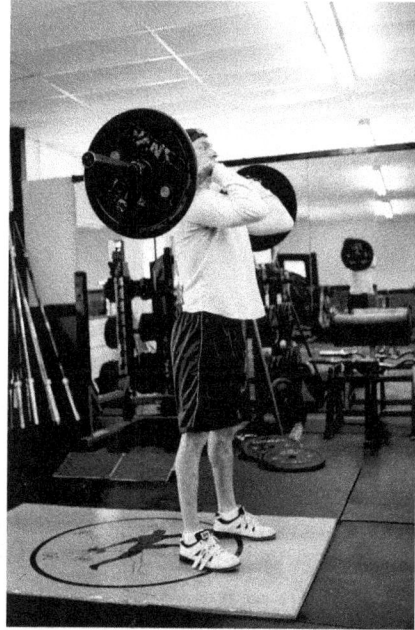

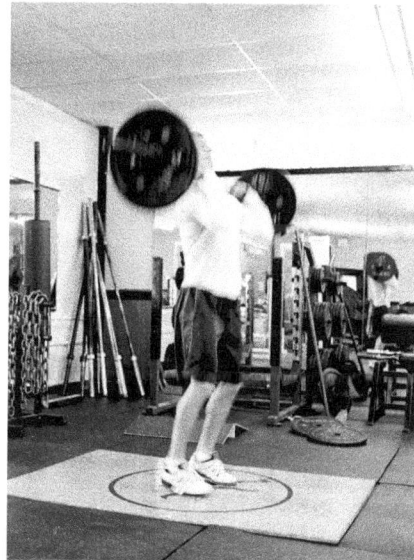

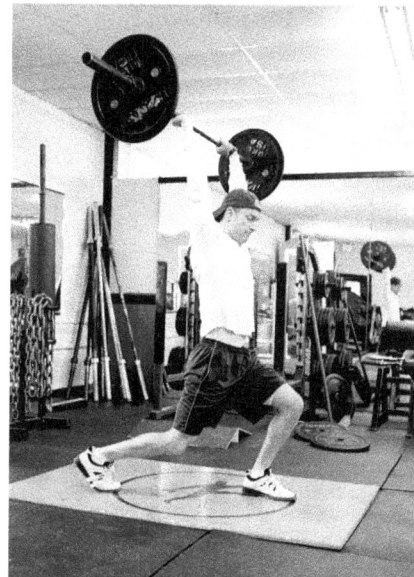

Push Press

Classification: Upper Body Press

Exercise Prerequisites: Avoid if you have persistent neck, knee, or low back pain.

Movement: Stand with feet in hip width staggered stance or hip width parallel stance. Hold barbell with pronated grip (palms forward). Begin with your upper arms pointing downward/slightly forward with triceps making contact with lats. The barbell should rest on the front anterior deltoid and upper chest musculature. Keeping the pelvis neutral, heels in contact with the floor, torso rigid, and eyes straight, explosively bend knees 10-20 degrees. Immediately reverse direction, driving through the legs and hips to generate momentum. Carry the momentum generated through the legs and hips and press the bar straight upward. Once the barbell has passed the top of your head, tuck your chin downward, gazing down at the ground roughly 5-10 feet in front of you (make sure not to hit your head with the bar). Continue pressing straight upward, until you have reached full extension of the arms and shoulders. Try to bring your shoulders to ear height at the top of the movement. Once you reach top position, slowly lower back to start.

Keys to Movement:
1. Keep torso upright throughout entire movement.
2. Hold barbell in pronated grip.
3. Triceps in contact with lats at the beginning of the movement.
4. Quick knee bend, followed by extension to generate momentum from the legs and hips.
5. Tuck your chin once the barbell has passed the top of your head.
6. Do not allow your back to arch as you press overhead.
7. "Active" shoulders at the top.

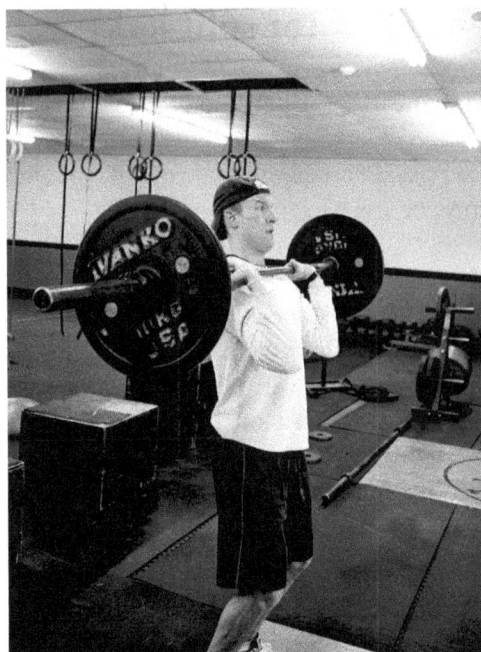

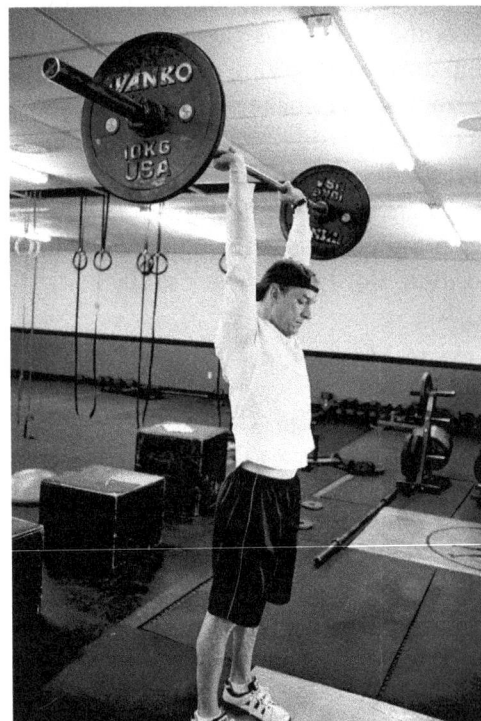

Rack Pull

Classification: Posterior Chain Extensor

Exercise Prerequisites: Avoid if you have neck, knee, or low back pain or lack flexibility to assume proper starting position.

Movement: Pronated grip is preferred for higher repetitions while mixed grip may be preferred for lower reps. It is very important to begin the rack pull in the proper starting position as the mechanics and success of the movement depend heavily on this initial body positioning. Position a barbell across safety pins at roughly knee or upper shin height. Begin by creating a lordotic posture in the spine, with chest out, shoulder pulled back, eyes straight ahead. Lean the torso over to roughly 45 degrees and walk your shins to the bar or 1 inch away from the bar. Keeping the angle of the torso relative to the floor, begin bending at the knees in order to grasp the bar. Keep the weight shifted to the heels (you should be able to wiggle your toes in the start position). Once your body positioning is correct begin the lift by pulling the shoulders up first, trying to maintain torso angle and rigidity. Do not raise the hips first as this can put excessive strain on your low back ligaments. As you raise, focus on pulling the bar toward you, clearing your knees so the bar can travel in as straight a line as possible. Extend the hips and knees, increasing the torso angle, until the bar comes in contact with the bottom part of the upper thigh. Once you have reached complete extension of the hips and knees, retrace the movement pattern during the eccentric part of the movement.

Keys to movement:

1. Proper start position is imperative.
2. Roughly 45 degree of torso relative to ground.
3. Bar in contact with shins or one inch away in starting position.
4. Back arched with weight through the heels.
5. Mixed grip for low reps and pronated grip for higher reps.
6. Focus on raising the shoulders first, keeping the same angle at the torso throughout the movement.
7. Do not raise the hips first.
8. At the top of the movement, do not lean back.
9. Retrace the same movement pattern during the eccentric part of the movement.

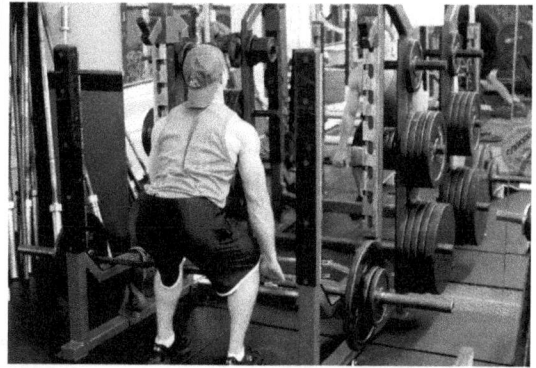

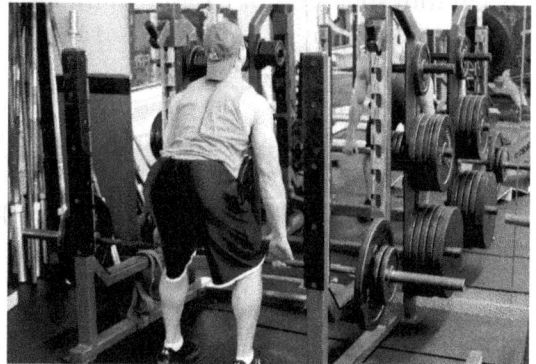

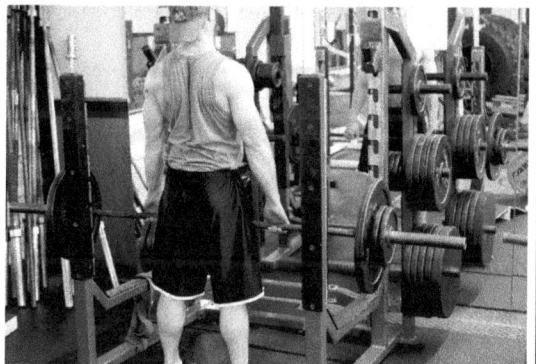

Reverse Hyperextension

Classification: Posterior Chain Extensor

Exercise Prerequisites: Avoid if you have excessive chronic or acute low back pain.

Antagonistic Muscles to movement: Hip flexors

Movement: Lay down on a reverse hyperextension machine. Begin with your feet down toward the floor with legs straight. Initiate the movement from the glutes and hamstrings, pulling your feet upward toward the ceiling. Pull to the point where your legs are parallel to the floor or your low back begins to lose neutral posture. Contract your glutes at the top of the movement and lower slowly and perform again. Once you finish with one leg, then perform desired repetitions for the opposite leg.

Keys to Movement:

1. Keep hips flat on the pad Do not allow rotation at the pelvis or low back.
2. Keep legs straight and initiate movement from the glutes and hamstrings.
3. Extend hips up to the point where legs are parallel to the floor or you lose posture in your low back.
4. Contract glutes at the top.
5. You can adjust foot positioning for different hamstring musculature emphasis.

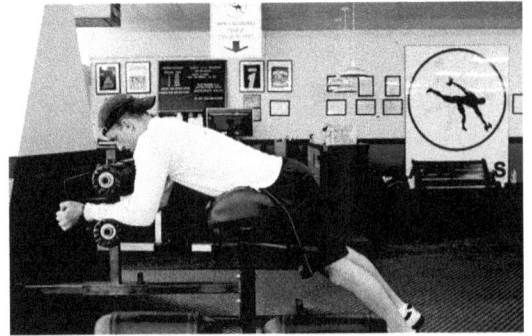

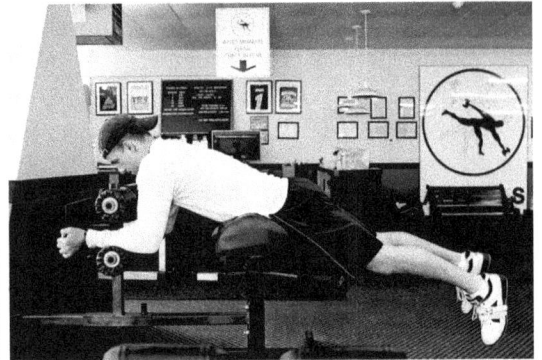

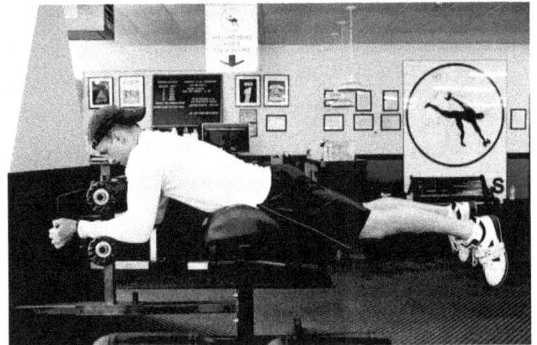

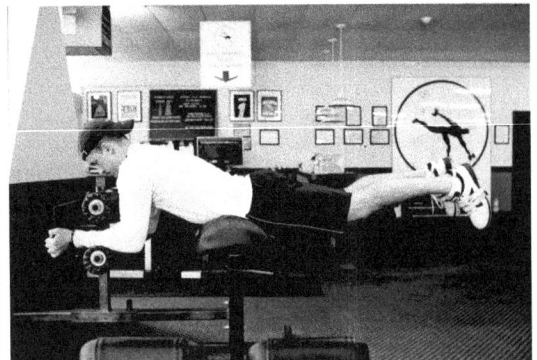

Ring Inverted Row

Classification: Upper Posterior Chain Pull Movement

Target Muscles: Trapezius, Latissimus Dorsi, Rhomboids, Rear Delts, Posterior Rotator Cuff Muscles, Low Back Extensor Chain

Exercise Prerequisites: Correct activation of glutes, hamstrings, low back extensors, rear deltoids, lats, and rhomboids. Avoid if you have persistent, low back, elbow, or shoulder pain

Antagonistic Muscles to movement: Shoulder internal rotators and elbow extensors.

Movement: With hands roughly shoulder width apart, grasp a set of rings with pronated or neutral grip. Lay on your back with your (heels) resting on the floor or on a Swiss ball. Extend hips and push chest out so body is in neutral/slightly lordotic posture. Maintaining posture, pull chest upward to the rings, initiating movement by retracting the shoulder blades and driving the elbows back. Once your chest makes contact with the rings, slowly lower back to start without breaking posture.

Keys to Movement:

1. Grasp the rings with pronated or neutral grip and hands slightly wider than shoulder width.
2. Extend hips and keep back in lordotic/neutral posture.
3. Do not allow hips to flex throughout movement.
4. Retract shoulder blades and pull chest to the rings.
5. Lower back to start position.

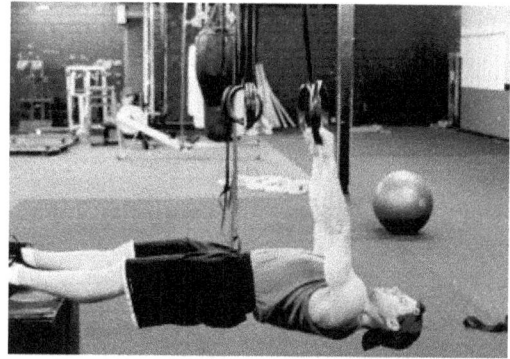

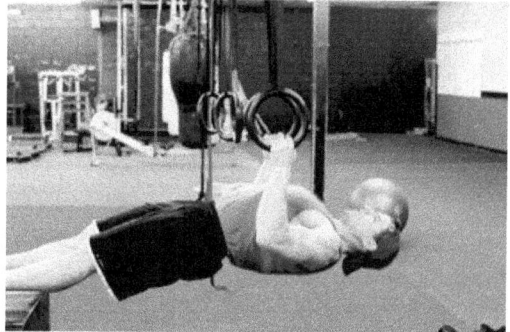

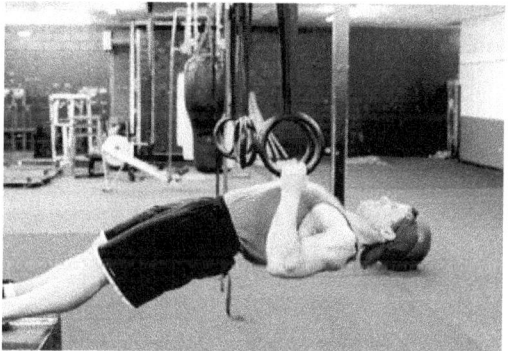

Ring Pushups

Classification: Upper Body Push

Target Muscles: Pectorals, Anterior Deltoids, Triceps, Rectus Abdominus, Obliques, TVA

Exercise Prerequisites: No shoulder pain. 20 Perfect form Pushups. If upper crossed syndrome is an issue, perform corrective movements prior to bench pressing.

Movement: Position your body into pushup position with hand on rings and feet hip width or closer. Your hands should be directly below your shoulders, with palms facing each other in neutral grip. Create intra-abdominal pressure to stabilize the pelvis and spine and squeeze glutes to deactivate hip flexors. Slowly lower body keeping neutral posture in torso, until your chest is parallel to your hands. To minimize shoulder problems, your elbows should be at a 45 degree angle or less relative to your torso. Make sure to keep your head looking down and your hips locked. Raise body back to start position, keeping locked into neutral posture.

Keys to Movement:

1. Body rigid with glutes squeezed and head looking down.
2. Keep elbows at 45 degrees or less relative to the torso.
3. Maintain neutral grip throughout movement.
4. Lower until hands are parallel to chest.
5. Never allow the hips to dip downward during the movement.

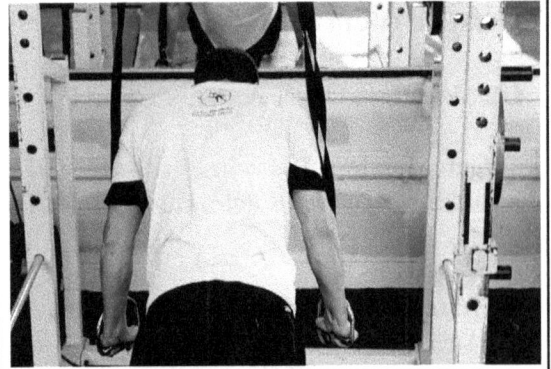

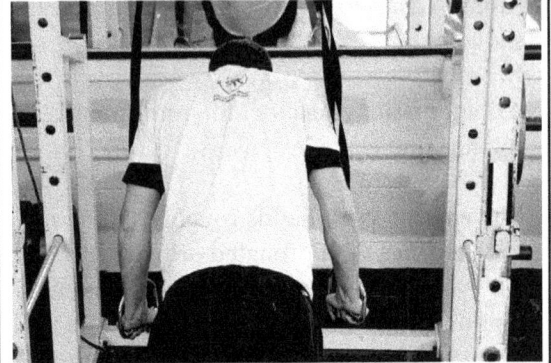

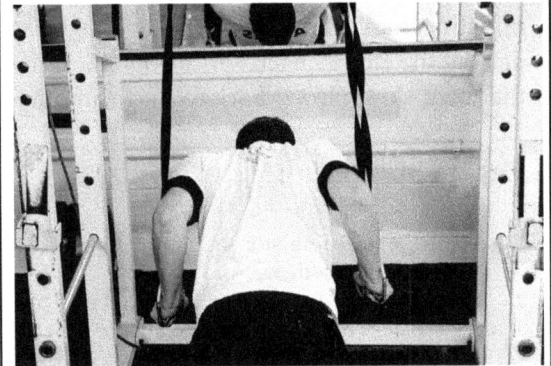

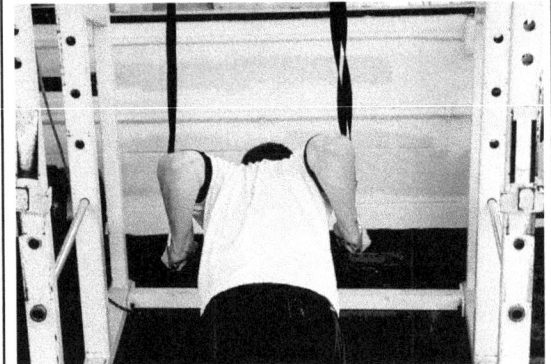

Romanian Deadlift

Classification: Bilateral Posterior Chain Extensor

Exercise Prerequisites: Avoid if you have persistent knee, neck, or low back pain.

Movement: It is very important to begin with a proper starting position, because the mechanics and success of the movement depend heavily on the body positioning at the beginning. Stand in front of a barbell with your feet parallel and roughly shoulder width apart. Position your torso into a lordotic posture, with chest out, shoulder pulled back, eyes straight ahead, and knee bent 20 degrees with hips higher than the knees. Keep the weight distributed over the rear of the foot. Begin by bending at the waist to ensure the muscle tension is created in the glutes and hamstrings, rather than the low back. Lean over by bending at the hips only keeping the knees locked at 20 degree angles. The upward pull is initiated through the glutes and hamstrings, while keeping the upper torso angle the same. You begin by pulling your squeezed scapula upward and back, extending the hips, increasing the torso angle, and bringing the bar back up to the start position until the torso is erect with a high chest posture. Once at the top position, slowly lower the barbell focusing on maintaining the exact same knee flexion angle and back arch. Lower to the point where your hamstrings a feeling a good stretch. The knee bend should remain the same throughout the movement. This is another exercise that is posterior chain specific, not lower back specific. As a matter of fact, if you feel it more in your lower back than glutes and hamstrings you may be doing it wrong.

Keys to Movement:
1. Knees bent roughly 20 degrees with feet hip width apart.
2. Back arched with weight shifted toward the heels.
3. Bend at the hips only, keeping knees locked at roughly 20 degree angle.
4. Think "big butt" when you are driving upward.
5. Lower to point in which you can longer maintain lordotic posture.

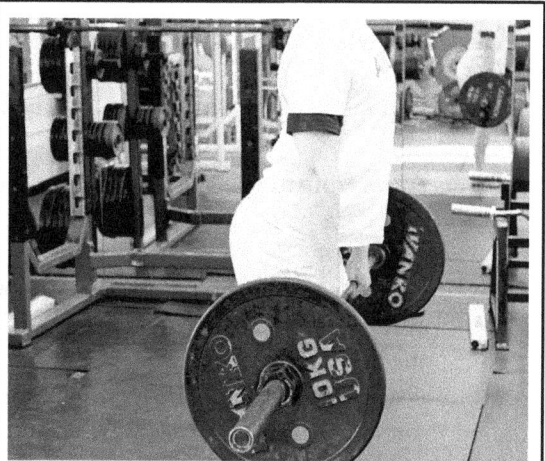

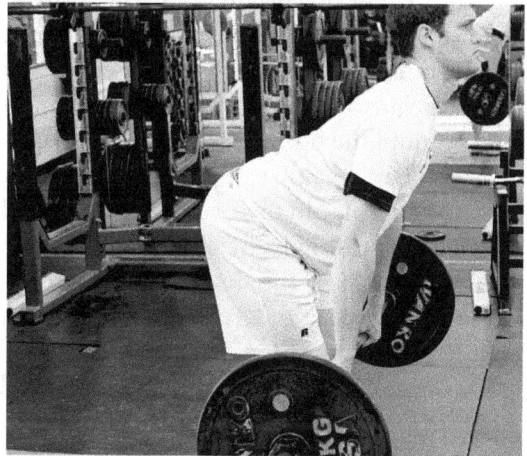

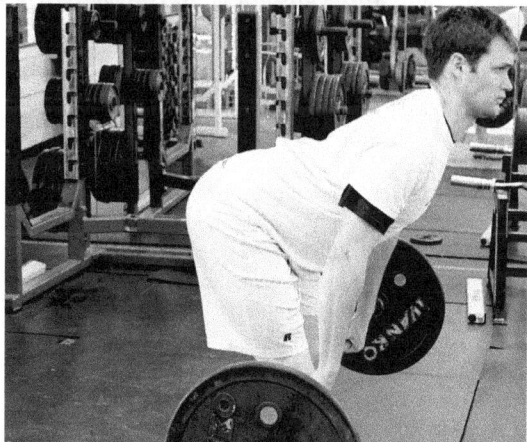

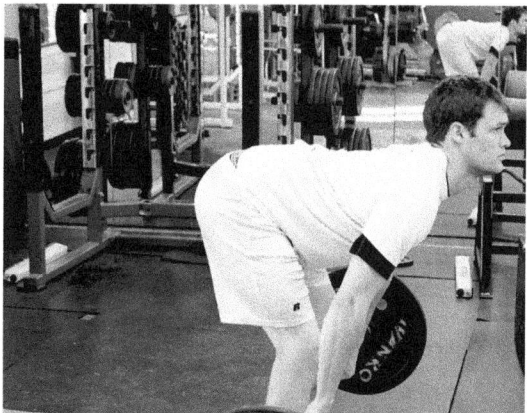

Rotational Low Back Extension

Classification: Posterior Chain and knee Extensor

Exercise Prerequisites: Avoid if you have persistent neck, knee, or low back pain.

Movement: Set up on either 45 degree or conventional back extension machine, with the Achilles tendon pressed firmly against the foot pad. With forearms crossed and hands on opposite shoulders, maintain lordotic/neutral posture and begin lowering your torso. At the same time, begin rotating opposite elbow downward toward opposite knee, maintaining back posture throughout. At the bottom, the upper body should be rotated with opposite side elbow across the body. The ascent begins with extension and "un-winding" of the torso. Extend until the body is in neutral starting position. Perform reps on one side, rest, and perform reps for the opposite side. To add resistance to this exercise, use a dowel stick across the upper back with light weight loaded on one side only. Once you progress past the dowel, move onto light barbells and eventually proceed to Olympic barbell. A dumbbell can also be used to enhance the effect of this exercise. As you rotate downward, reach toward the ground below the opposite side knee. During the concentric motion, perform a dumbbell row at the same time, ending up in full isometric contraction with your torso parallel to the floor at the top.

Keys to Movement:
1. Position body in correct start position on conventional back extension machine.
2. Lower down, rotating opposite elbow toward opposite side knee.
3. At the bottom, the upper body should be rotated with opposite side elbow across the body.
4. Raise up by uncoiling and extending at the same time until you reach neutral starting position.
5. Do not hyperextend.

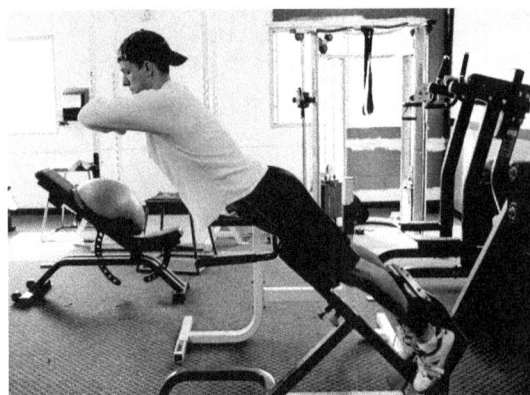

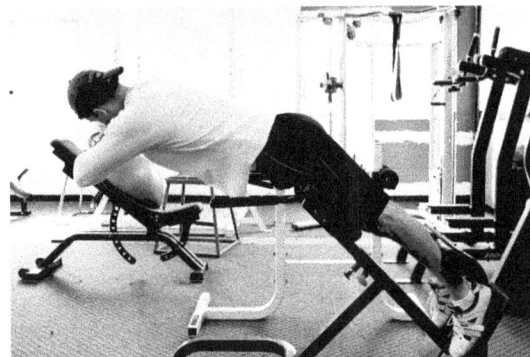

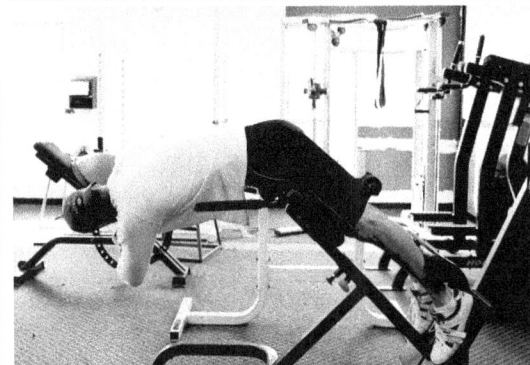

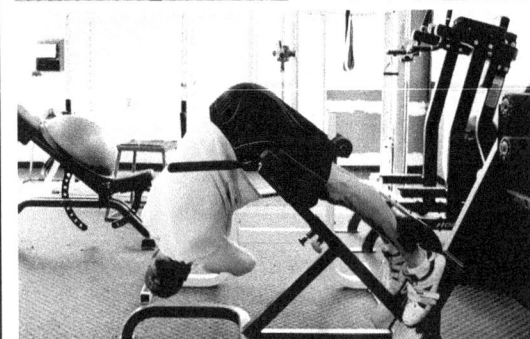

Rotational Plank

Classification: Low Back, Core, Rotational Mechanics

Target Muscles: Low Back, Core, Rotary Musculature

Exercise Prerequisites: Avoid if you have persistent, low back, neck, or shoulder pain

Movement: Position yourself in a conventional plank position but with your forearms parallel to each other and feet spread wider than the hips. Keeping the body locked, with neutral spine, begin the movement by sliding your left elbow laterally, placing all of the weight on your right elbow and feet. Make sure your hip does not move or rotate prior to the elbow movement. After you have slid the elbow laterally, begin rotating the hips, torso and feet at the same time, while driving the left elbow up and backward as you rotate. You should end up in a position similar to a side plank. Rotate the body back to the start position with both elbows on the floor and do the same movement pattern on the opposite side.

Movement Mechanics:

1. Position in conventional plank position, but with forearms parallel to each other and perpendicular to the body.
2. Shift weight to one forearm without moving hip.
3. Begin rotation at the elbow prior to hip moving
4. Rotate all the way until hip and shoulder are parallel to a wall
5. Lower back to start position and perform on other side.

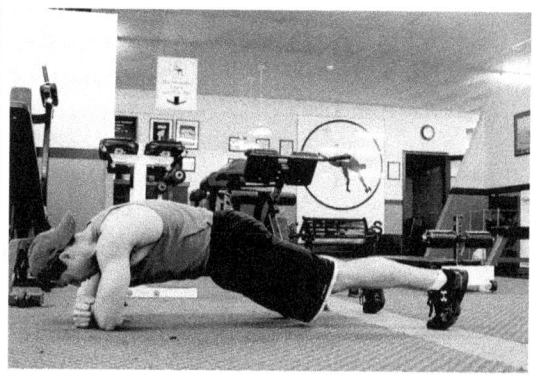

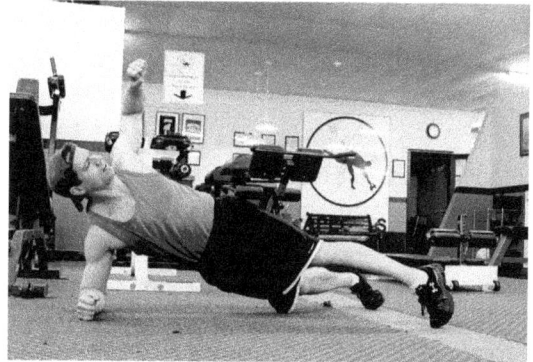

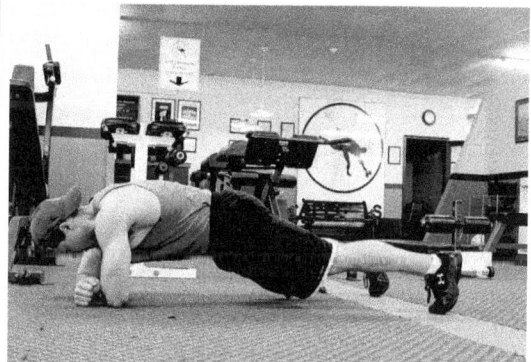

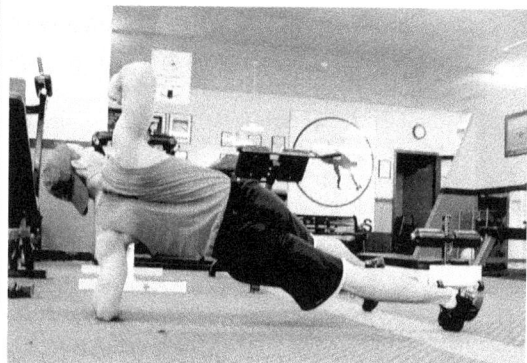

Seated Cable Row

Classification: Upper Posterior Chain Pull Movement

Target Muscles: Trapezius, Latissimus Dorsi, Rhomboids, Rear Delts, Posterior Rotator Cuff Muscles, Low Back Extensor Chain, glutes, quads, hamstrings, tibialis anterior

Exercise Prerequisites: Correct activation of rear deltoids, rhomboids, and latissimus musculature. Avoid movement if you have low back pain

Antagonistic Muscles to movement: Shoulder internal rotators, elbow extensors.

Movement: Sit on a seated cable row machine facing the row handle. Holding the cable handle in front of the body, begin by bending the knees approximately 20 degrees. Arch your back into a lordotic posture, with chest out, shoulder pulled back and down, eyes straight ahead. Ensure that your shoulders/torso remains directly over the hips as there is a tendency to lean back during the rowing movement.

Pull the weight toward your sternum/belly button, activating first the rear delt muscles, then pulling with the larger rhomboid and lat muscles. To do this, retract your shoulder blades back and down, then focus on pulling back with the elbows until full contraction of the upper back musculature. Ensure not to allow the shoulders to shrug upward as this takes away from the contraction of the mid back/shoulder retractor muscles. Make sure there is no bounce or rounding of the back throughout the movement. Slowly lower the weight back to start and perform next repetition.

Movement Mechanics:

1. Position body in correct starting position with knees bent 20 degrees, chest out, back arched, and shoulder directly over hips.
2. Initiate movement by retracting shoulders back and down, maintaining shoulders directly over hips.
3. Focus on pulling elbows back.
4. Do not allow shoulders to shrug upward.
5. Do not lean torso backward.
6. Row back until complete contraction of shoulder blades.

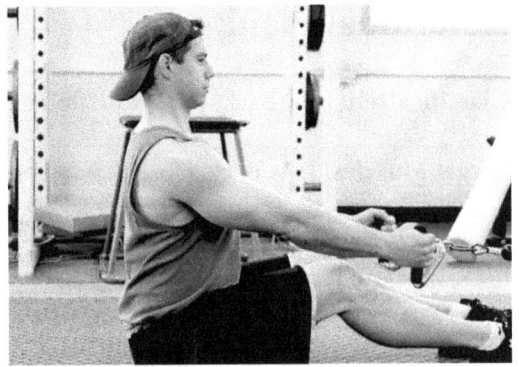

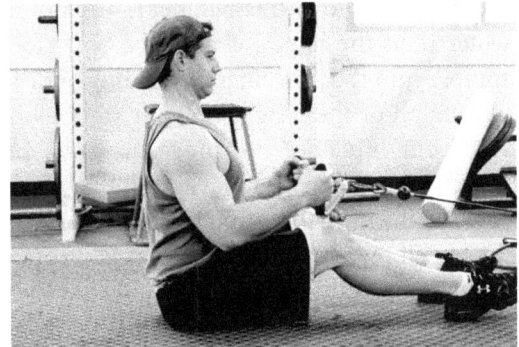

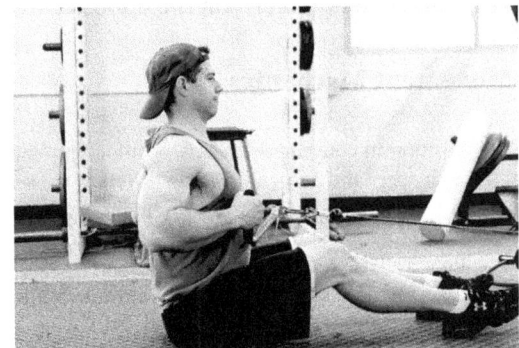

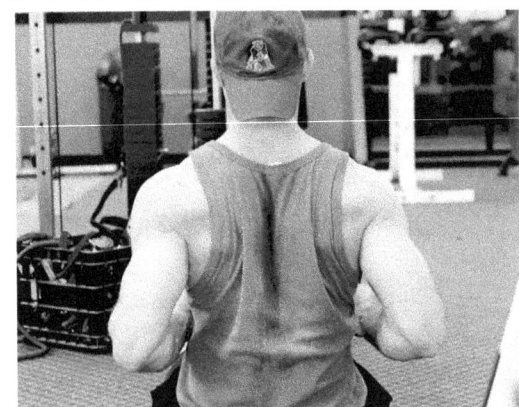

Seated Dumbbell External Rotator

Classification: External Rotator

Exercise Prerequisites: Avoid if you have persistent neck, shoulder or low back pain.

Movement: Sit on a bench with one foot on the bench and the other foot on the floor with knees bent. Holding a dumbbell in the hand of the foot on the bench hand, place your elbow on your knee. Focus on keeping a 90 degree angle at the elbow throughout the entire movement. Lower the dumbbell down toward the inside of your thigh by internally rotating at the shoulder. Once in a bottom position, externally rotate upward back to start position. Ensure that you keep the elbow in contact with knee throughout the movement.

Keys to Movement:

1. Keep torso upright throughout entire movement.
2. Ideally, you should have a 90 degree angle at the hips when positioning for the exercise.
3. Same side elbow on top of the knee that is on the bench.
4. Keep elbow in contact with knee throughout the movement.
5. Maintain 90 degree angle throughout movement.

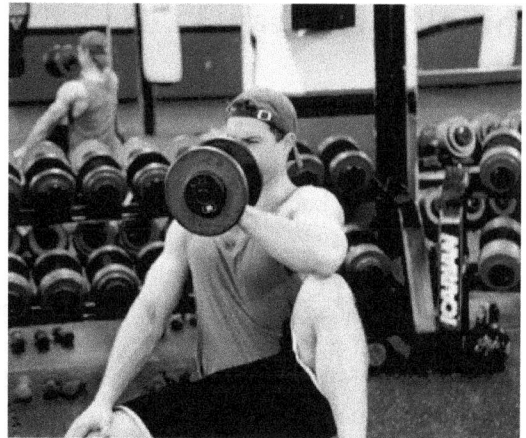

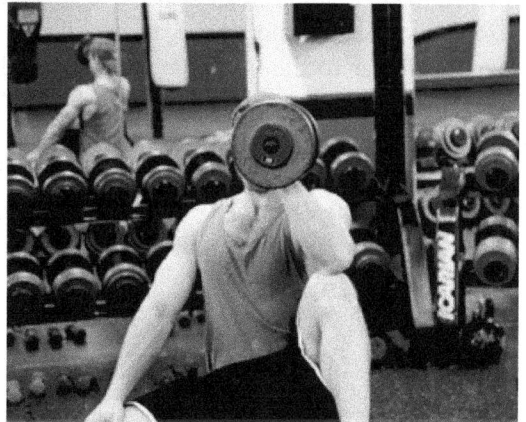

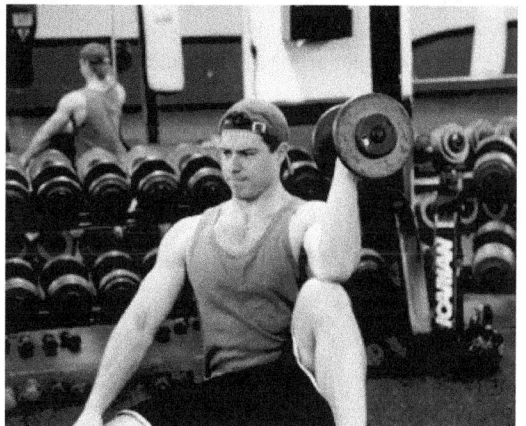

Single Arm Trap-3 Lift

Classification: Scapular Structural Balance

Exercise Prerequisites: Avoid if you have persistent neck, shoulder or low back pain.

Movement: Hold a dumbbell in one hand with thumb pointing upward. Your other arm should rest forearm across a stable object with your torso at a 45 degree angle. Rest your forehead on the forearm that is braced. Position your feet in a staggered stance, left foot back and right foot forward, slightly behind you. Maintaining a neutral or slightly arched posture, extend your arm holding the dumbbell downward until it is perpendicular to the floor. Retract the shoulder blade of the arm holding the dumbbell down and back. With the scapular retraction, raise the extended left arm at a 45 degree angle away from the head until the elbow passes the ear. Once the elbow passes the ear, reach outward and lower back to start.

Keys to Movement:

1. Torso at a 45 degree angle to the floor with forearm resting against a brace.
2. Feet staggered with foot on the side of the hand holding the dumbbell back.
3. Retract shoulder blade keeping arm straight to start the movement.
4. Raise straight arm at 45 degree angle from the head until the elbow passes the ear.
5. Reach away as you lower.

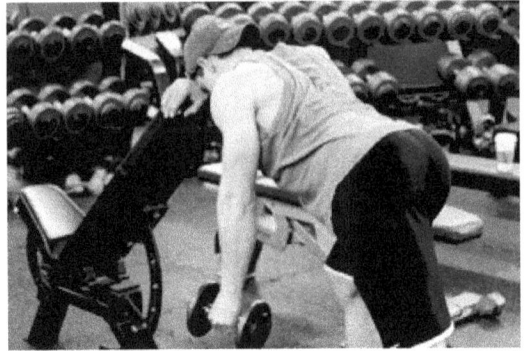

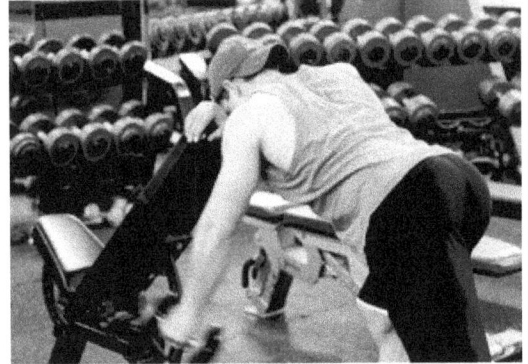

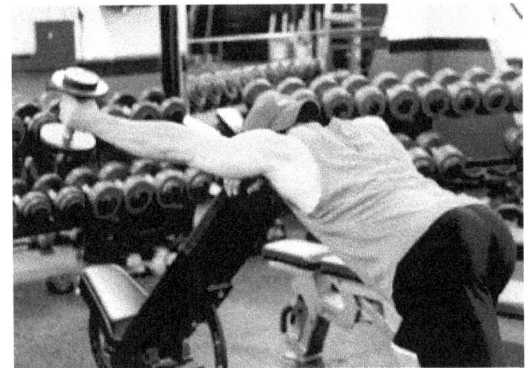

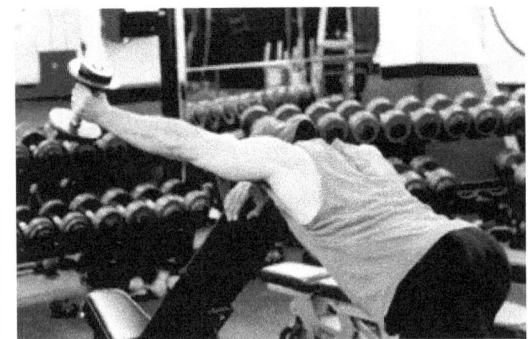

Side Bridge or Side Lying Oblique

Classification: Low Back and Core

Exercise Prerequisites: Avoid if you have persistent knee, shoulder, neck, or low back pain.

Movement: As back problems are associated with the law enforcement profession, unilateral strengthening of the quadratus lumborum and synergistic recruitment of the oblique musculature can aid in creating a healthy low back. Compressive loading resistance exercises including squats and deadlifts could potentially exacerbate any asymmetrical imbalances of the low back musculature. Conventional low back extension variations may not correct the imbalance as the overactive musculature may be preferentially recruited. The side lying bridge, a favorite of world renowned low back specialist Dr. Stuart McGill, and the side lying oblique are two exercises that put emphasis on the oblique and Quadratus Lumborum musculature unilaterally. These exercises can be highly practical for repairing and maintaining optimal low back health in law enforcement professionals.

Lie on your side with your hand or elbow on a padded surface. With your legs and feet stacked, lift your hips off the ground, maintaining contact with the ground on your elbow/hand and feet only. Make sure to keep the hips completely extended and glutes contracted to provide proper activation of the QL and abdominal musculature.

Keys to Movement:

1. Lie on your side with hand or elbow on padded surface.
2. With legs and feet stacked, raise your hips straight upward.
3. Do not allow your top hip to rotate backward.

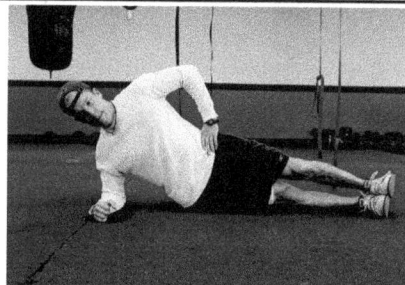

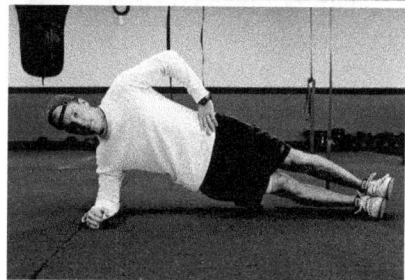

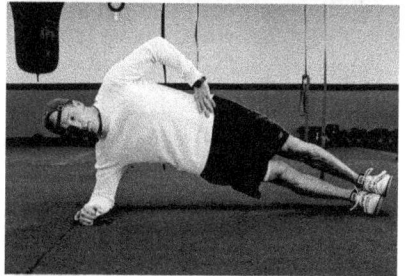

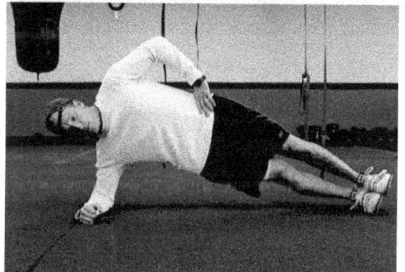

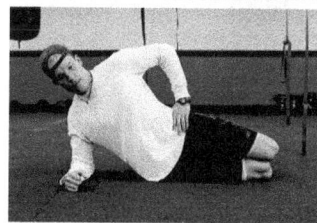

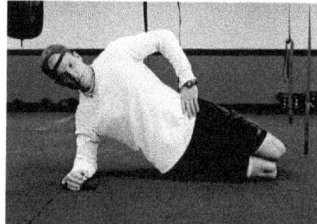

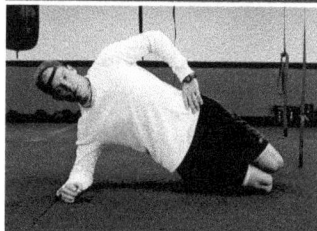

Snatch Variations

Classification: Upper Posterior Chain Pull Movement

Target Muscles: Trapezius, Latissimus Dorsi, Rhomboids, Levator Scapulae, Brachialis, Biceps Brachii

Exercise Prerequisites: Correct activation of Latissimus Dorsi and rhomboids. Do not do if you have elbow, shoulder or serious low back pain

Antagonistic Muscles to movement: Internal rotators, elbow extensors

Movement: Grasp a pull-up bar with hands pronated, shoulder width or slightly wider. Hang from the bar, with arms, hips and shoulders in complete extension. Initiate movement by retracting shoulder blades back and down. Begin pulling your body straight upward, continuing to pull the shoulder blades back and downward. Do not allow the shoulder to internally rotate as you are pulling upward.

Pull upward, pinching your shoulder blades back until the upper portion of the chest comes in contact with the bar.

Lower the body slowly, retracing the same pattern until you reach full extension starting position at the bottom.

If you cannot perform a regular pull-up, you can use the assistance of a partner or a band around the knee or foot.

Keys to Movement:

1. Pronated grip with hands shoulder width or slightly wider.
2. Begin in "dead hang" position.
3. Retract shoulders back and down prior to and during the movement.
4. Focus on pulling the elbows back and down.
5. Do not allow the shoulders to internally rotate,
6. Pull up until upper part of chest comes in contact with the bar.
7. Lower down until full extension in the elbows and shoulders.

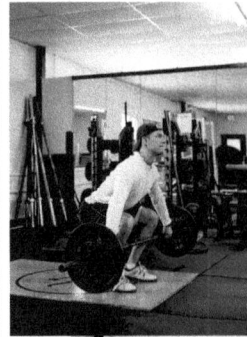

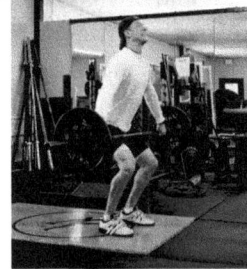

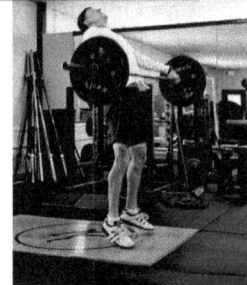

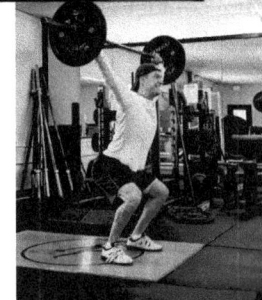

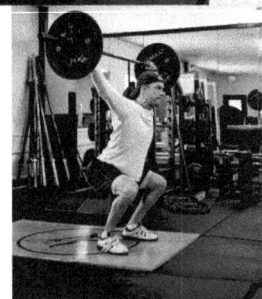

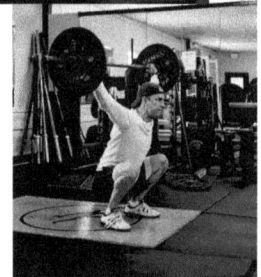

Split Squat Jumps

Classification: Sub maximal Plyometric

Exercise Prerequisites: Avoid if you have chronic knee, ankle, or low back problems.

Movement: Position body into bottom part of a lunge. Maintain torso in upright position with knees and feet pointing straight ahead. Drive straight up as high as you can off both legs, initiating movement from front leg hips extensor musculature. Once you have reached peak jump height, scissor kick legs and land softly with opposite leg in front position. Dip back down in to lunge and jump, emphasizing lead leg hip extensors. Try to make sure you are on the ground no longer than 1 second, with .3-.7 seconds being ideal.

Keys to Movement:

1. Position legs into correct lunge position with torso in rigid upright position.
2. Feet and knees pointing straight ahead.
3. Focus on driving through lead leg hip extensors.
4. Keep hip square. Do not allow them to rotate throughout the movement.
5. Minimal ground contact time between jumps.

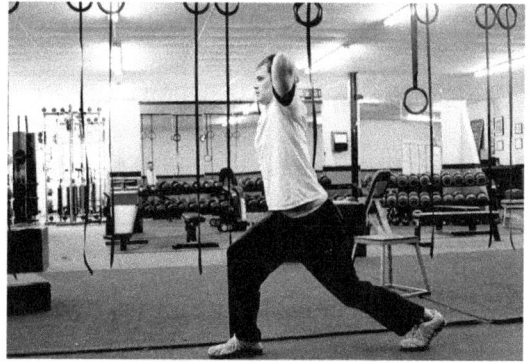

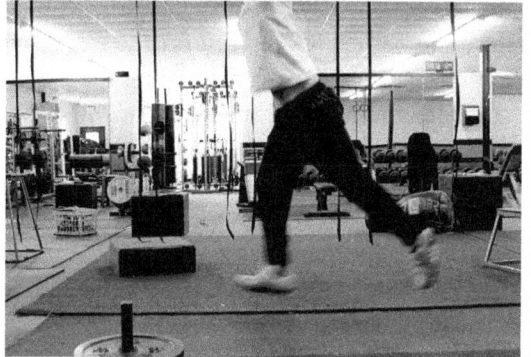

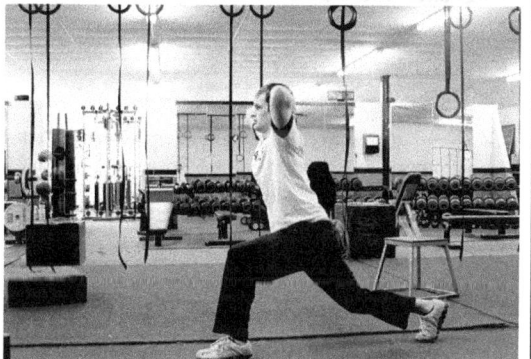

Standing Barbell Overhead Press

Classification: Upper Body Press

Exercise Prerequisites: Avoid if you have persistent neck, knee, or low back pain.

Movement: Stand with feet in hip width staggered stance or hip width parallel stance. Hold dumbbells with pronated grip (palms forward). Begin with your upper arms pointing downward/slightly forward with triceps making contact with lats. The barbell should rest on the front anterior deltoid and upper chest musculature. Keeping the pelvis neutral, heels in contact with the floor, and eyes straight, begin pressing straight upward. Once the barbell has passed the top of your head, tuck your chin downward, gazing down at the ground roughly 5-10 feet in front of you (make sure not to hit your head with the bar). Continue pressing straight upward, until you have reached full extension of the arms and shoulders. Try to bring your shoulders to ear height at the top of the movement. Once you reach top position, slowly lower back to start.

Keys to Movement:

1. Keep torso upright throughout entire movement.
2. Do not allow heels to come off the ground.
3. Hold barbell in pronated grip.
4. Triceps in contact with lats at the beginning of the movement.
5. Tuck your chin once the barbell has passed the top of your head.
6. Do not allow your back to arch as you press overhead.
7. "Active" shoulders at the top.

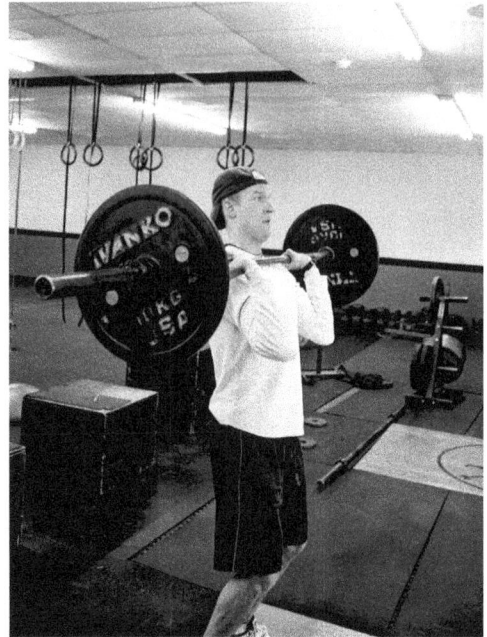

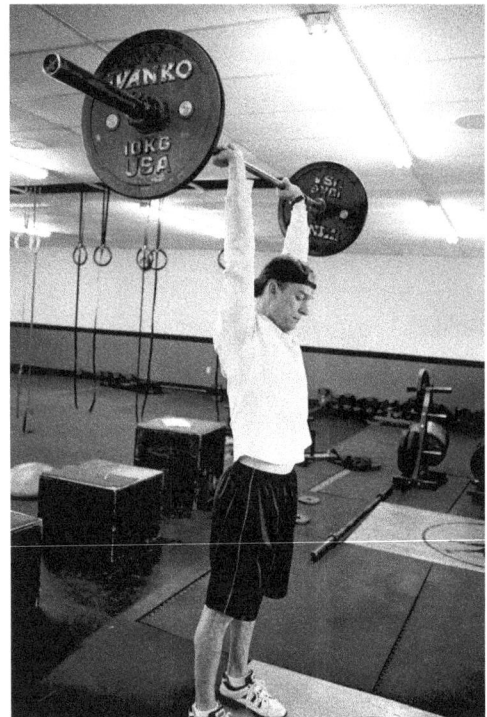

Standing Cable External Rotator

Classification: External Rotator

Exercise Prerequisites: Avoid if you have persistent neck, shoulder or low back pain.

Movement: Stand next to a cable column with your upper arm down by your side and elbow bent 90 degrees. Make sure the elbow is kept directly below the shoulder capsule throughout the movement. If it is allowed to abduct or adduct, the recruitment of the external rotator musculature can be altered. Keeping the upper arm locked in place, begin externally rotating the humerus, maintaining the 90 degree angle at the elbow. The forearm is kept parallel to the floor throughout the movement. Rotate as far as your muscles/flexibility allows or until your break technique or elbow angle.

Keys to Movement:

1. Keep torso upright throughout entire movement.
2. Elbow is directly below the shoulder capsule. Do not actively adduct or abduct.
3. Maintain 90 degree angle at the elbow throughout the movement.

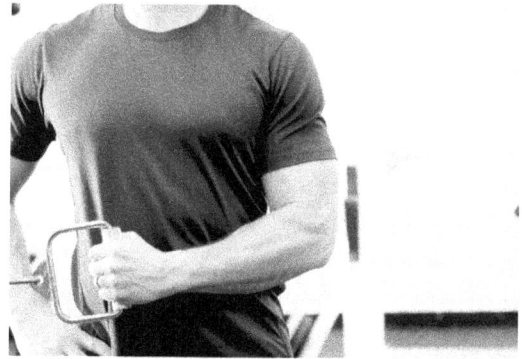

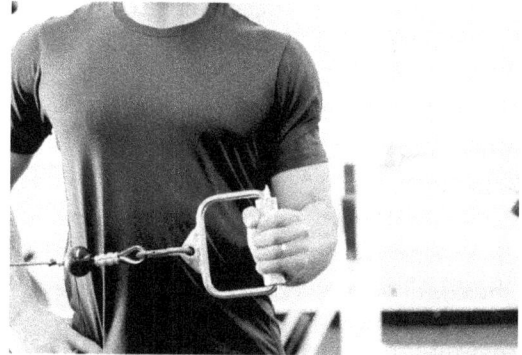

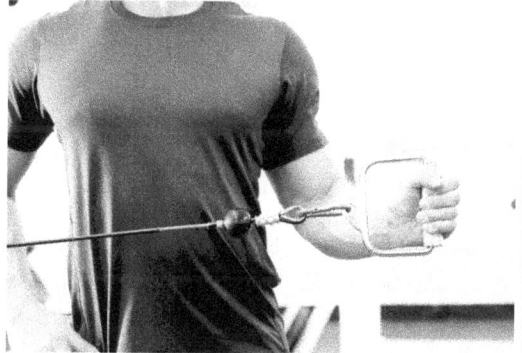

Standing Dumbbell Overhead Press

Classification: Upper Body Press

Exercise Prerequisites: Avoid if you have persistent neck, knee, or low back pain.

Movement: Stand with feet in hip width staggered stance or hip width parallel stance. Hold dumbbells with neutral grip (palms together). Begin with your upper arms pointing downward with triceps making contact with lats. The dumbbells should be over or slightly in front of the anterior deltoid. Keeping the pelvis neutral, heels in contact with the floor, and eyes straight, begin pressing straight upward. Once the dumbbells have passed the top of your head, tuck your chin downward, gazing down at the ground roughly 5-10 feet in front of you. Continue pressing straight upward, until you have reached full extension of the arms and shoulders. Try to bring your shoulders to ear height at the top of the movement. Once you reach top position, slowly lower back to start.

Keys to Movement:

1. Keep torso upright throughout entire movement.
2. Do not allow heels to come off the ground.
3. Hold dumbbells in neutral grip throughout movement.
4. Triceps in contact with lats at the beginning of the movement.
5. Tuck your chin once the dumbbell has passed the top of your head.
6. Do not allow your back to arch as you press overhead.
7. "Active" shoulders at the top.

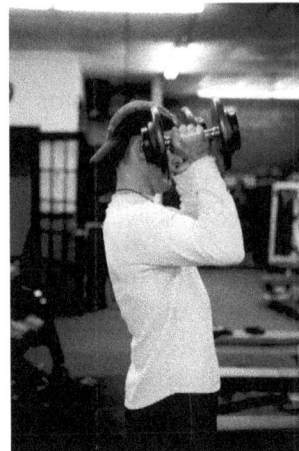

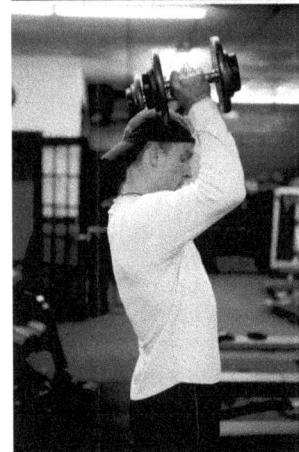

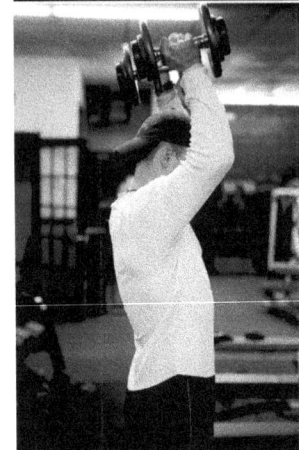

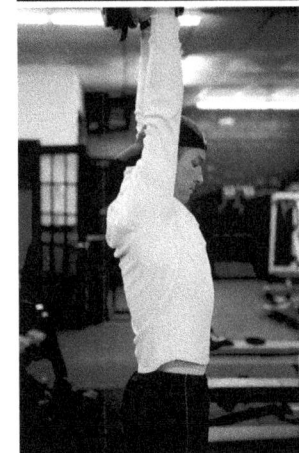

Standing Face Pull

Classification: Scap Retractor

Exercise Prerequisites: Avoid if you have persistent elbow, shoulder, neck, or low back pain.

Movement: Adjust a cable column to roughly shoulder/chin height. Attach a triceps rope to a cable column. Stand roughly three feet from the column with feet staggered. Grasp rope with pronated grip, arms extended and thumbs pointing toward the cable column. With arms parallel to the floor, begin by retracting the shoulder blades first. Initiate pull by pulling the elbows back and upward. Ensure that the elbows are higher than the hands throughout the movement. Pull back until your elbows are parallel to or behind your ears.

Keys to Movement:

1. Stand with feet staggered facing cable column.
2. Pronated grip on rope with thumbs forward.
3. Retract shoulder blades back first, then pull elbows backward.
4. Maintain elbows higher than hands.
5. Keep elbows above ear height when pulling back.
6. Pull back until elbows are parallel to or behind ears.

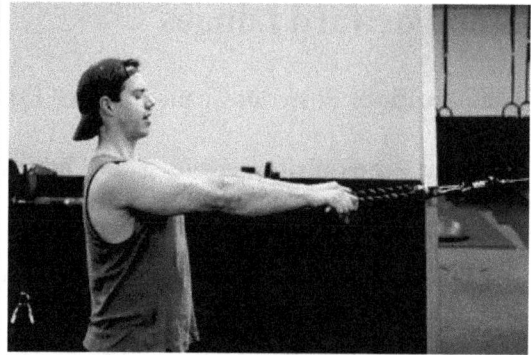

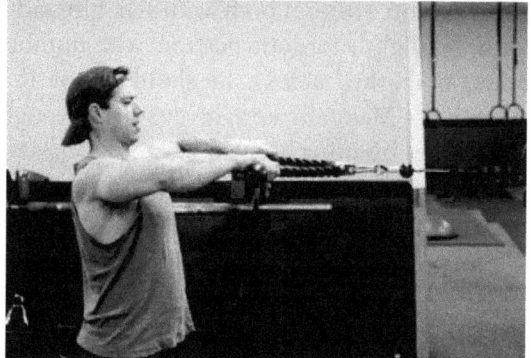

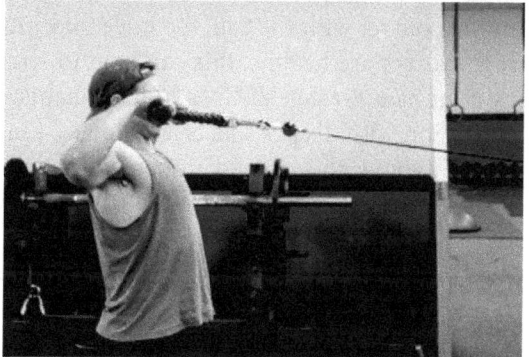

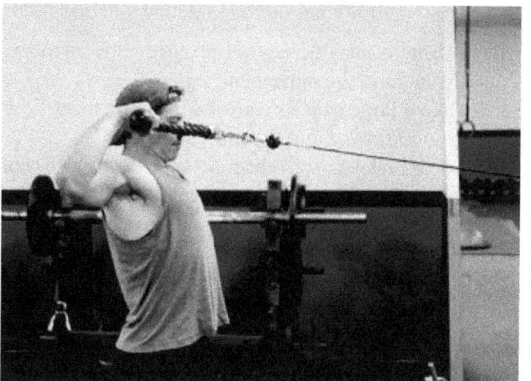

Step Forward Lunges

Classification: Posterior Chain and knee Extensor

Exercise Prerequisites: Avoid if you have persistent neck, knee, or low back pain.

Antagonistic Muscles to movement: Hamstrings as flexors of the knee.

Movement: Position body with feet hip width apart, torso in neutral/slightly lordotic posture, with dumbbells held at your sides or barbell across the shoulders or in font squat rack position. Maintain upright posture throughout movement. With toes pointing straight ahead, take a large step forward. Lower the hips forward and toward the ground maintaining upright posture with no lean forward. Keeping the back leg as straight as possible, descend until the hamstring comes in contact with the calf on the front leg. It is imperative not to lean forward or allow the front foot heel to come off the ground throughout the movement. As the hamstring comes in the contact with the calf, the knee may cross the toe plane. If the knees are healthy, this can help to strengthen the knee as there is a greater VMO, adductor, hamstring, and gluteal activation with deeper squats and lunges. Once the back knee is 1-2" above the ground initiate the backward movement through the ball of the front foot by driving the shoulders back to the start position with no change in posture. Perform all reps on one leg, then perform on the opposite leg.

Keys to Movement:

1. Maintain lordotic/neutral posture with torso perpendicular to floor throughout the movement.
2. Take a large step forward keeping the front heel in contact with the ground throughout the movement.
3. Focus on keeping the back leg as straight as possible to ensure maximal tension on front leg and stretching of back leg hip flexor musculature.
4. Lower down until hamstring comes in contact with calf. In health knees, the knee may cross of the toe plane as there is a greater recruitment of VMO, adductor, hamstring, and gluteal musculature.
5. Begin ascent by focusing on driving the shoulders/torso back and upward first.
6. Do not allow the front heel to come off during the movement.
7. Do not allow torso to lean over during the movement.

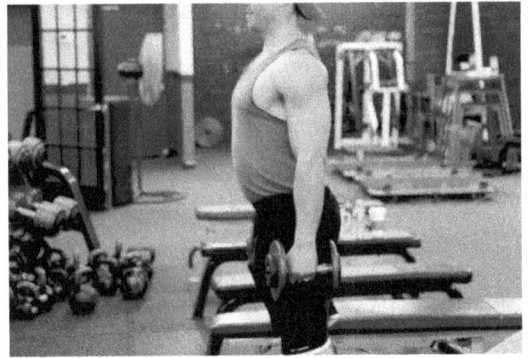

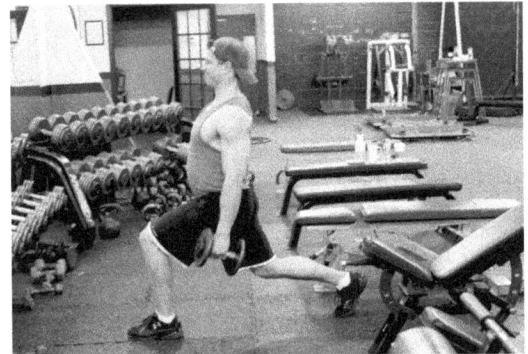

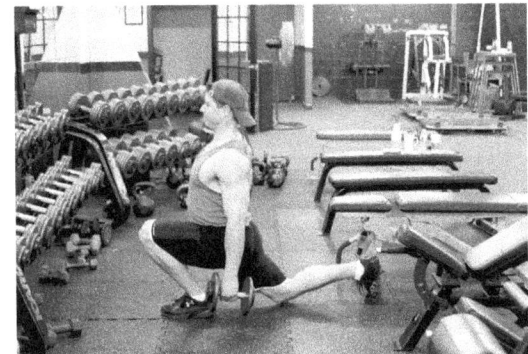

Suitcase Carries

Classification: Low Back and Core

Exercise Prerequisites: Avoid if you have persistent knee, shoulder, neck, or low back pain.

Movement: Similar to the asymmetrically loaded deadlift, lift the weight, keeping the torso locked upright, and walk X distance. Try not to allow the torso to lean forward or toward the weighted side. After you have completed your predetermined distance, perform on the alternate side.

Keys to Movement:

1. Keep torso in rigid neutral/lordotic posture, and lift weight on one side of the body with proper deadlift technique.
2. Keep torso upright. Do not allow torso to deviate toward either side.
3. Walk set distance.

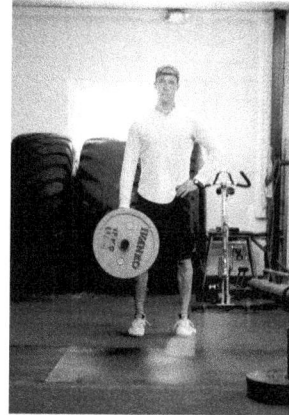

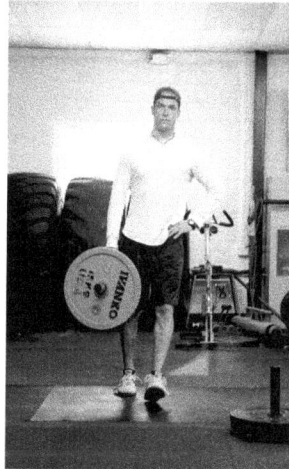

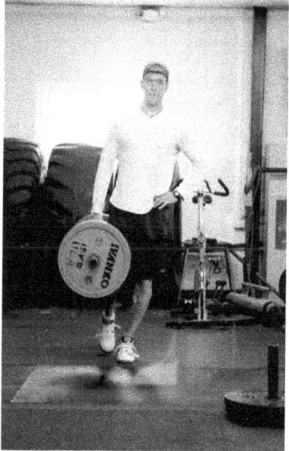

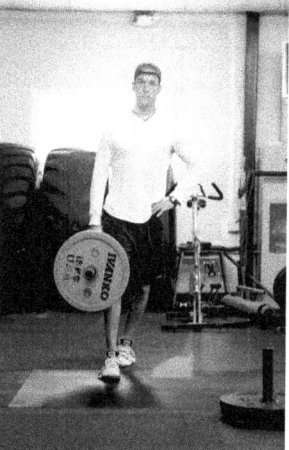

Swiss Ball Hamstring Curls

Classification: Posterior Chain and knee flexor

Exercise Prerequisites: Avoid if you have persistent neck, knee, or low back pain.

Antagonistic Muscles to movement: Knee Extensors, Hip Flexors

Movement: Lie flat on your back with your heels hip width apart on the top of a Swiss ball. Position your hands down by your sides with arms straight. Begin by bridging the hips (extending the hips) upward, maintaining shoulders in contact with the ground. Keeping a straight line between the shoulders, hips, and knees, begin curling your heels toward your glutes. The ball will roll toward your glutes as you do this. Once you have reached full flexion of the hamstrings, begin to lower slowly back to start. To correct structural imbalances about the hamstrings, you can adjust foot positioning by pointing the toes inward, outward, or neutral. Another option is to plantar flex the foot to minimize gastroc assistance.

Keys to Movement:

1. Lie flat on your back with heels hip width apart on top of a Swiss ball.
2. Extend hips, bringing glutes off the ground.
3. Make sure you have a straight line between shoulders, hips, and knees throughout the entire movement.
4. Curl heels toward your glutes.
5. Adjusting foot positioning can aid in correcting structural imbalances about the hamstring musculature.

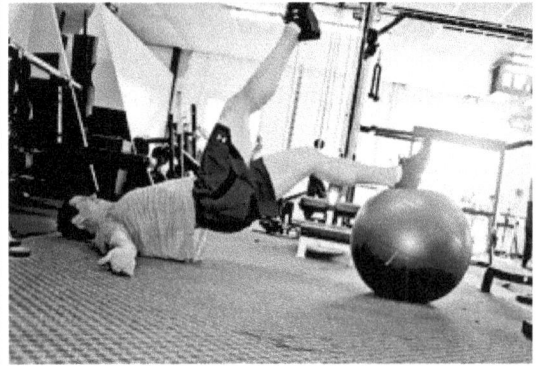

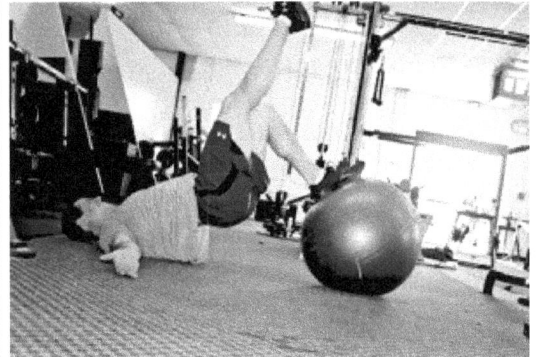

Swiss Ball Stir the Pot

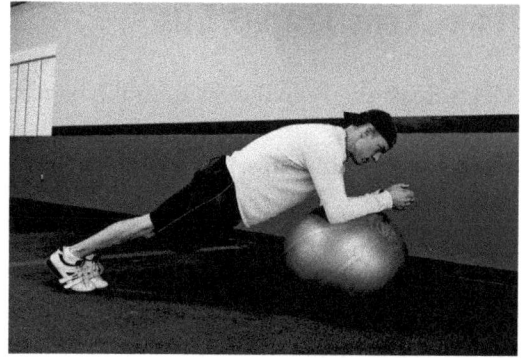

Classification: Low Back and Core

Exercise Prerequisites: Avoid if you have persistent knee, shoulder, neck, or low back pain.

Movement: Position your elbows on a Swiss ball with feet on the floor and body locked into a plank position. Contract your glutes and quads and begin "stirring the pot" or drawing out the letters of the alphabet with your elbows. Stop as soon as you feel stress or strain on the low back or once there is a breakdown in the quality of movement.

Keys to Movement:

1. With elbows directly below your shoulder on a Swiss ball, lock your body into rigid neutral position with glutes contracted.
2. Move elbows in "stirring the pot" fashion or draw letters of the alphabet with your elbows.

Two Arm Trap-3 Lift

Classification: Scapular Structural Balance

Exercise Prerequisites: Avoid if you have persistent neck, shoulder or low back pain.

Movement: Lie face down on a 45 degree incline bench with your chin resting on the top of the bench. Hold dumbbells in your hands with thumb pointing upward. Maintaining a neutral or slightly arched posture, extend your arms holding the dumbbell downward until it is perpendicular to the floor. Retract the shoulder blades down and back. With the scapular retraction, raise extended arms at a 45 degree angle away from the head until the elbows pass the ears. Once the elbows pass the ears, reach outward and lower back to start.

Keys to Movement:

1. Lie face down on a 45 degree incline bench.
2. Retract shoulder blades keeping arms straight to start the movement.
3. Raise straight arms at 45 degree angle from the head until the elbows pass the ears.
4. Reach away as you lower.

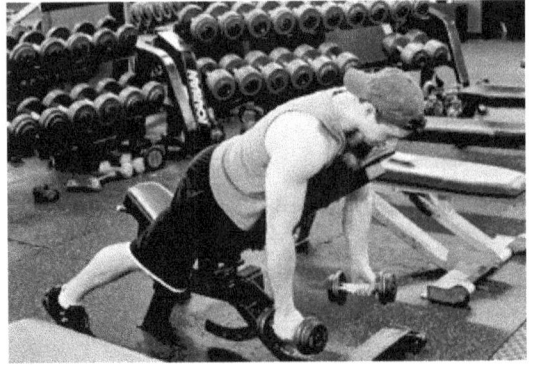

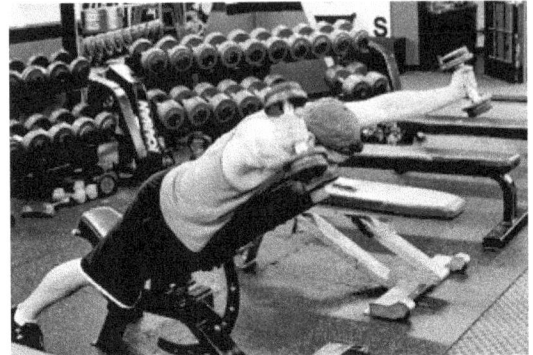

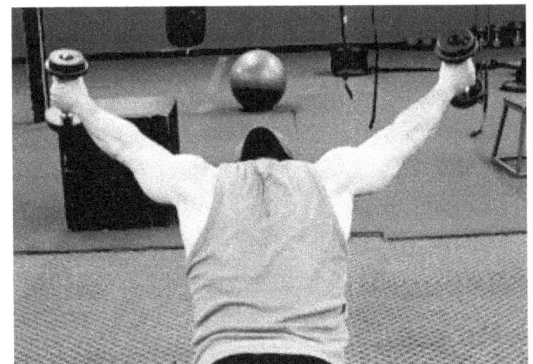

Walking Lunges

Classification: Posterior Chain and knee Extensor

Exercise Prerequisites: Avoid if you have persistent neck, knee, or low back pain.

Antagonistic Muscles to movement: Hamstrings as flexors of the knee.

Movement: Position body with feet hip width apart, torso in neutral/slightly lordotic posture, with dumbbells held at your sides or barbell across the shoulders or in font squat rack position. Maintain upright posture throughout movement. With toes pointing straight ahead, take a large step forward. Lower the hips forward and toward the ground maintaining upright posture with no lean forward. Keeping the back leg as straight as possible, descend until the hamstring comes in contact with the calf on the front leg. It is imperative not to lean forward or allow the front foot heel to come off the ground throughout the movement. As the hamstring comes in the contact with the calf, the knee may cross the toe plane. If the knees are healthy, this can help to strengthen the knee as there is a greater VMO, adductor, hamstring, and gluteal activation with deeper squats and lunges. Once the back knee is 1-2" above the ground initiate the upward/forward drive with the front foot heel, pulling the body forward and up into the original start position without the non-ground contact foot touching the ground until the next step. Keep the torso upright throughout the entire movement. Perform the same for the other leg, driving the knee and lunging forward, performing in a cyclic walking pattern.

Keys to Movement:

1. Keep torso upright throughout entire movement.
2. Do not allow front foot heel to come off the ground.
3. Keep lunging knee pointing in the same direction and lunge foot toes.
4. If the knees are health, lunge down and forward until hamstring touches the calf.
5. Try to keep back leg as straight as possible placing emphasis on lead leg.

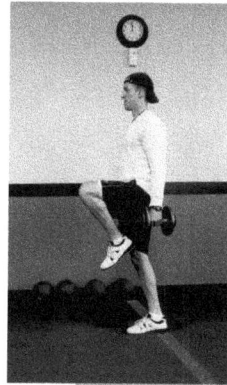

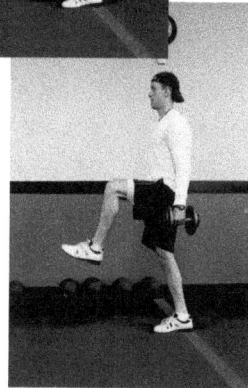

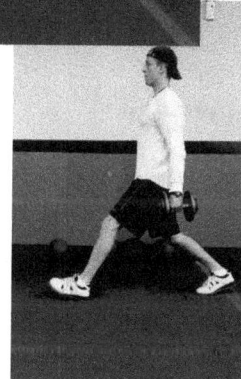

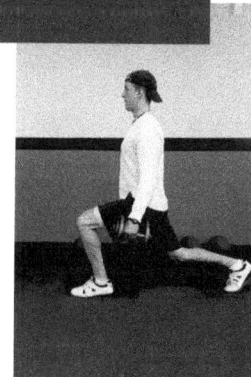

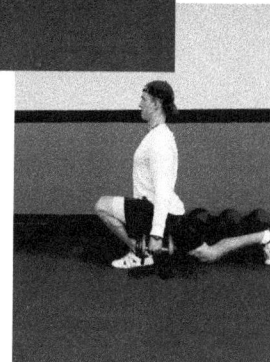

Wall Facing Squat

Classification: Lower body hip and knee extensor, hip mobility

Exercise Prerequisites: Glute, Hamstring, and Adductor activation. Avoid if chronic knee or low back pain.

Antagonistic Muscles to movement: Hamstrings as flexors of the knee.

Movement: Stand with toes against a wall in a conventional squat starting position. Toes pointing outward about 15-20 degrees. With your hands on top of your head and begin to squat. Allow your knees to touch the wall and squat as low as you can, maintaining weight on the heels and feet against the wall. Be careful not to fall backward. A spotter with hand placed in the middle of the back can aid in increasing range of motion without risk of falling. Ensure that the knees point in the same direction as the toes throughout the entire movement.

Keys to Movement:

1. Stand with toes touching the wall, pointing outward 15-20 degrees.
2. Ensure that the knees point in the same direction as the toes as you squat down.
3. Allow the knees to touch the wall first.
4. Squat as low as you can, maintaining posture and technique.
5. A spotter with hand placed in middle of the back can aid in increasing range of motion without falling over.
6. Keep heels in contact with the ground throughout the movement.

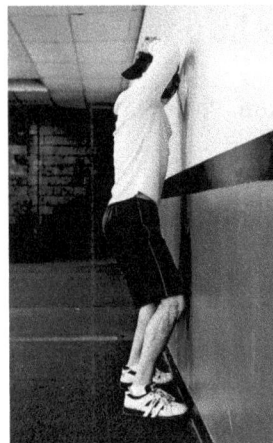

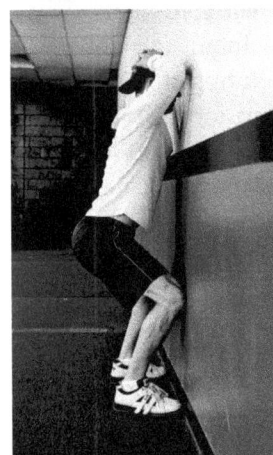

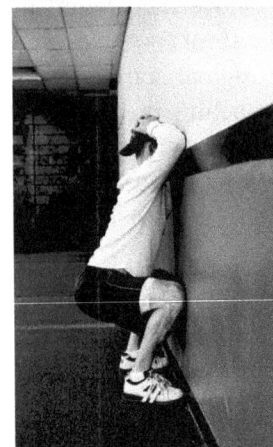

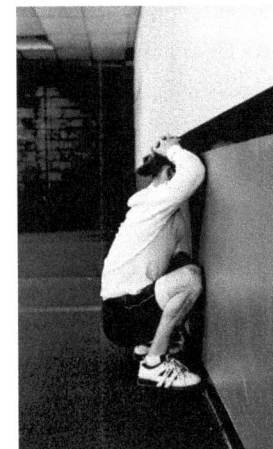

Wall Series

Classification: Shoulder Prehab

Exercise Prerequisites: Avoid if you have persistent shoulder, neck pain.

Movement: Sit with your back and butt flat against a wall, with your legs in butterfly stretch position. Start by holding a dowel rod just above your head, with elbows pressed firmly against the wall bent at 90 degree angles. Keeping your butt, back, and head flat against the wall, begin pressing the dowel rod overhead, making sure to keep your elbows and hands in contact with the wall. Perform for 10-15 reps.

The second exercise in the wall series begins in the same position as above, but this time you will rotate the dowel rod down toward your chest while keeping the upper arms parallel to the floor. Once you reach your chest, rotate the dowel rod back to the wall.

Keys to Movement:

1. Sit with your butt and back flat against the wall.
2. 90 degree angle at elbows with hands and elbows against the wall
3. Press overhead maintaining contact with elbows and hands with the wall.

1. Same start position.
2. Keep upper arm parallel to the floor.
3. Maintain contact with elbows and upper arms against the wall.
4. Rotate down toward chest.
5. Rotate upward over head until hand return to the wall.

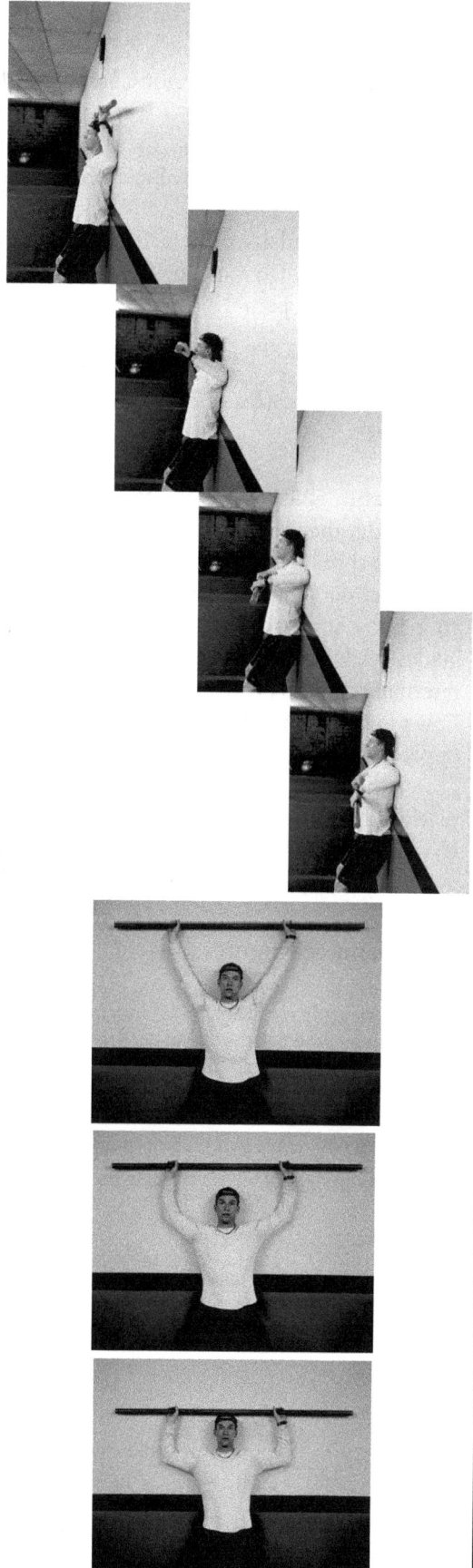

Wide Pull-ups

Classification: Upper Posterior Chain Pull Movement

Target Muscles: Trapezius, Latissimus Dorsi, Rhomboids, Levator Scapulae, Brachialis, Biceps Brachii

Exercise Prerequisites: Correct activation of Latissimus Dorsi and rhomboids. Do not do if you have elbow, shoulder or serious low back pain

Antagonistic Muscles to movement: Internal rotators, elbow extensors

Movement: Grasp a pull-up bar with hands pronated, about 6-12' wider than the shoulders. Hang from the bar, with arms, hips and shoulders in complete extension. Initiate movement by retracting shoulder blades back and down. Begin pulling your body straight upward, continuing to pull the shoulder blades back and downward. Do not allow the shoulder to internally rotate as you are pulling upward.
Pull upward, pinching your shoulder blades back until the upper portion of the chest comes in contact with the bar.
Lower the body slowly, retracing the same pattern until you reach full extension starting position at the bottom.
If you cannot perform a regular pull-up, you can use the assistance of a partner or a band around the knee or foot.

Movement Mechanics:

1. Pronated grip with hands 6-12" wider than the shoulders.
2. Begin in "dead hang" position.
3. Retract shoulders back and down prior to and during the movement.
4. Focus on pulling the elbows back and down.
5. Do not allow the shoulders to internally rotate,
6. Pull up until upper part of chest comes in contact with the bar.
7. Lower down until full extension in the elbows and shoulders.

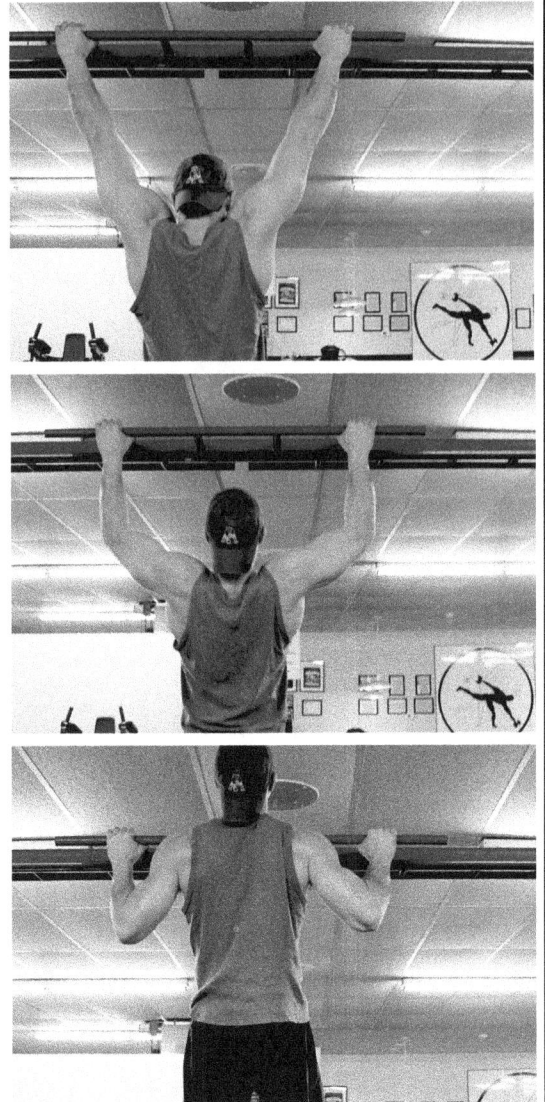

Windshield Wipers

Classification: Low Back and Core

Exercise Prerequisites: Avoid if you have persistent knee, shoulder, neck, or low back pain.

Movement: Lie flat on your back with arms anchored in a "T" position out to your sides. With your back flat on the floor, lift your legs until perpendicular to the floor, with feet above hips. A variation is to keep the knees bent at roughly 90 degrees with the lower leg parallel to the floor. Keeping your hips in contact with the floor, rotate at the hips, lowering the legs to the floor on one side. Rotate back to start, and then perform on the opposite side, similar to the movement of a "windshield wiper".

Keys to Movement:

1. Lie flat on your back with arms anchored in a "T" position.
2. Keep thighs perpendicular to the floor with knees bent or straight.
3. Rotate both knees as a unit down toward the floor on one side, keeping the opposite side shoulder in contact with the ground.
4. Rotate back to start.

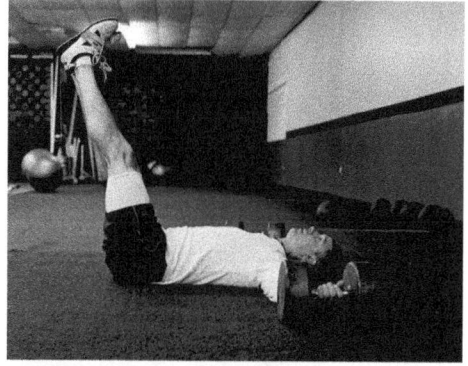

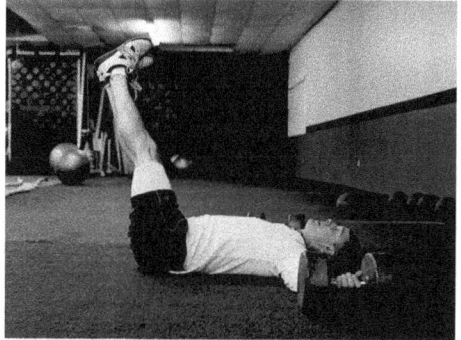

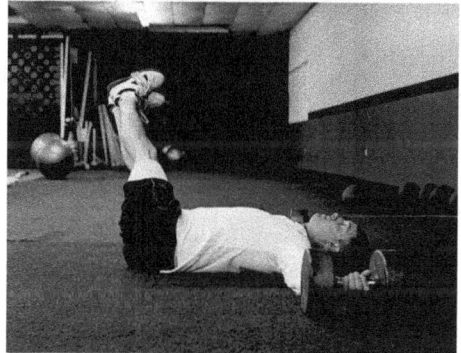

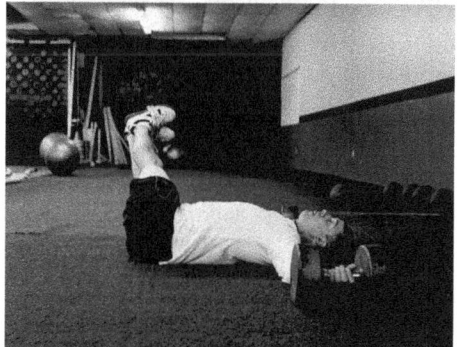

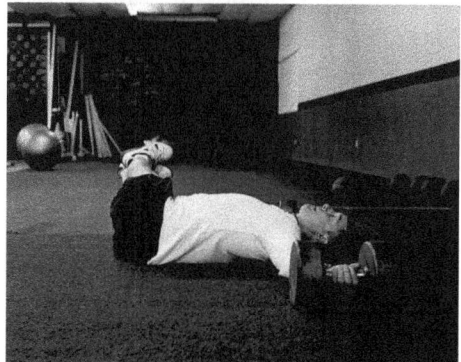

W, Y, T, L

Classification: External Rotators and Scapula Retractors

Exercise Prerequisites: Avoid if you have persistent shoulder, neck, or low back pain.

Movement: Lie face down on a bench. For each of these, picture looking down from the ceiling at the relative position of your arms to your body. The movement should draw parallels to the letter associated with the exercise.

W: Lie face down on a bench with your elbows directly by your sides, with forearms parallel to the floor at a 45 degree angle relative to your upper arm. Your thumbs should be pointing upward. Keeping your head down, externally rotate your upper arms, rotate your forearms upward, and squeeze your shoulder blades together, forming the letter W with your upper arms and forearms. Lower back to start.

Y: Lie face down on a bench with your arms at a 45 degree angle relative to your head extended over your head. With your thumbs pointing upward, retract your shoulder blades, and raise your extended arms until your elbows pass your ears. Ensure that your maintain the upper arms at a 45 degree angle relative to your head throughout the movement.

T: Lie face down on a bench with arms extended perpendicular to your body out to your sides. With your thumbs up, raise your arms from the floor, squeezing your shoulder blades until your upper arms are parallel to the floor. Ensure that your thumbs are pointing upward and extended arms are kept perpendicular to the body throughout the movement.

L: Lie face down on a bench with elbows bent 90 degrees and upper arms perpendicular to the shoulder capsule. The upper arms should be parallel to the floor, with a 90 degree angle at the armpit. The forearms are perpendicular to the floor at the start of the movement. Maintaining 90 degree angle at the elbows and armpit, externally rotate the upper arms, raising the forearms until they are parallel to the floor.

Keys to Movement:

1. Lie face down on a bench.
2. Focus on complete range of motion.
3. Watch for deviations in upper arm positioning relative to the torso.

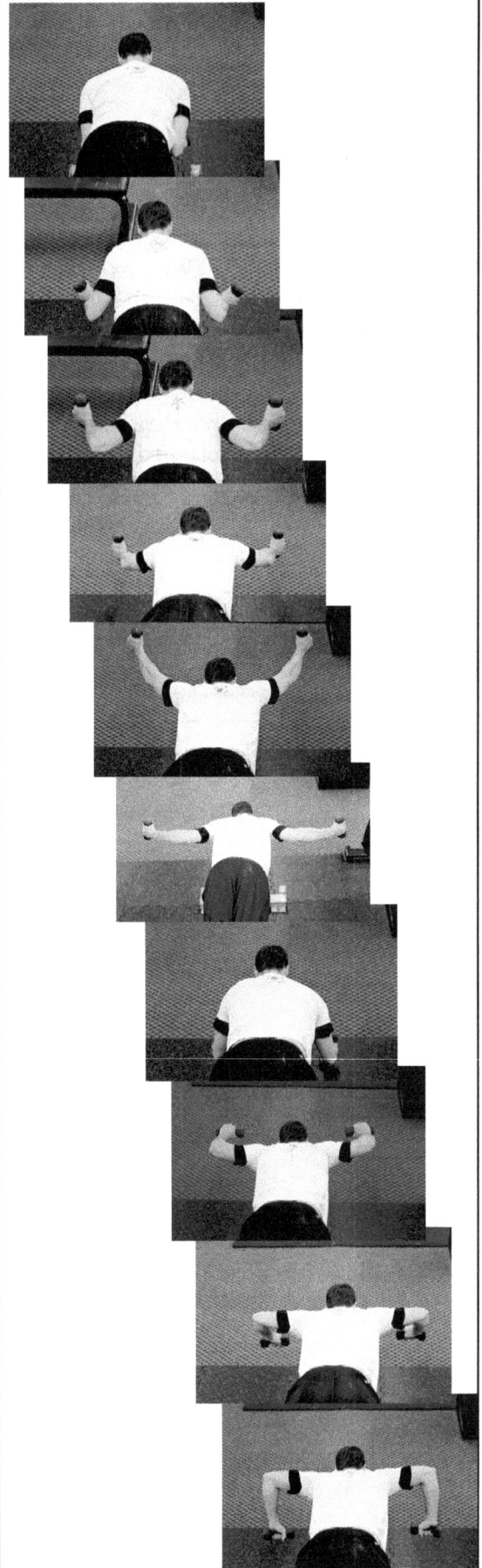

References

Chapter I

1. Bondarchuk A et al. **Adaptation.** *Soviet Sports Review.* 23(3); Pp 105-106. 1988

2. Cormie P, McCauliey G, Triplett N, Mcbride J. **Optimal loading for maximal power output during lower-body resistance exercises.** *Medicine and Science in Sports and Exercise.* 39(2); Pp 340-349. 2007.

3. Cormie P, Martin W, Bloomfield S, Lowry O, Holloszy J. **Effects of Detraining on Responses to Submaximal Exercise.** *Journal of Applied Physiology.* 59(3); Pp 853-859. 1985.

4. Coyle, E., Hemmert, M., Coggan, A. **Effects of Detraining on Cardiovascular Responses to Exercise: Role of Blood Volume.** *Journal of Applied Physiology* 60: Pp 95-98, 1986.

5. Dupont G., Akakpo K., Berthoin S., **The Effect of In-season, High Intensity Interval Training in Soccer Players.** *Journal of Strength and Conditioning Research,* 18(3): Pp584-589. 2004.

6. Fleck, S. **Detraining: Its Effects on Endurance and Strength.** *National Strength and Conditioning Association Journal. 16(1);* Pp 22-28. 1994.

7. Francis C., **Planning/Periodization;** *The Charlie Francis Training System.* Pp102. 1991.

8. Francis, C. **Recovery and Regeneration.** *The Charlie Francis Training System.* Pp61-86. 1991

9. Hakkinen, K, Komi, P. **Alterations of Mechanical Characteristics of Human Skeletal Muscle During Strength Training.** *European Journal of Applied Physiology.* 50; Pp 161-172. 1983.

10. Hakkinen K, Keskinen K. **Muscle Cross-Sectional Area and Voluntary Force Production Characteristics in Elite Strength and Endurance Trained Athletes and Sprinters.** *European Journal of Applied Physiology.* 59; Pp 215-220. 1989.

11. Hakkinen K, Pakarinen A, Alen M, Komi P. **Serum Hormones During Prolonged Training of Neuromuscular Performance.** *European Journal of Applied Physiology.* 53; Pp 287-293. 1985.

12. Hoffman J, Kang J. **Strength changes during an in-season resistance training program for football.** *Journal of Strength and Conditioning Research.* 17(1); Pp 109-114. 2003

13. Homenkova L. **Physical Training.** *Fitness and Sports Review International.* 29(3-4). Pp136-140. 1994

14. Hori N, Newton R, Andrews W, Kawamori N, Mcguigan M, Nosaka K. **Does performance of hang clean differentiate performance of jumping, sprinting, and change of direction.** *Journal of Strength and Conditioning Research.* 22(2); Pp 412-418. 2008

15. Hortobagyi, T, Houmard, J, Stevenson, J, Fraser,D, Johns, R, Israel, R. **The Effects of Detraining on Power Athletes.** *Medicine and Science in. Sports and Exercise.* 25; Pp 929-935. 1993

16. Jullien H, Bisch C, Largouet N, Manouvrier C, Carling C, Amilard V. **Does a short period of lower limb strength training improve performance in field based tests of running and agility in young professional soccer players?** *Journal of Strength and Conditioning Research.* 22(2); Pp 404-411. 2008

17. Kraemer et el. Detraining **Produces Minimal Changes in Physical Performance and Hormonal Variables in Recreationally Strength Trained Men.** *Journal of Strength and Conditioning Research.* 16(3); Pp 373-382. 2002.

18. Menkhin Y. **How to measure exercise loads.** *Fitness and Sports Review International.* 28(5-6); Pp 159-161. 1993.

19. Mosher M., Peterson D., **Effect of In-Season Training on Body Composition and Bench press Strength of Collegiate Women Track Sprinters.** *IAHPERD Journal,* 30 (2), 1997.

20. Mujika I, Padilla S. **Muscular Characteristics of Detraining in Humans.** *Medicine and Science in Sports and Exercise.* 33(8); Pp 1297-1303. 2001.

21. Mujika I, Padilla S. **Detraining: Loss of Training-Induced Physiological and Performance Adaptations. Part I.** *Sports Medicine.* 30(2); Pp 79-87. 2000.

22. Mujika I, Padilla S. **Detraining: Loss of Training-Induced Physiological and Performance Adaptations. Part II**. *Sports Medicine.* 30(3); Pp 145-154. 2000.

23. Neufer, D, Costill, D, Fielding, R, Glynn, and Kirwan, J. **Effect of Reduced Training on Muscular Strength and Endurance in Competitive Swimmers**. *Medicine and .Science in Sports and Exercise.* 19; Pp486-490. 1987

24. Nicholas S, Tyler T. **Adductor muscle strains in sport.** *Journal of Sports Medicine.* 32(5); Pp 339-344. 2002

25. Nunez V, Grigoletto M, Castillo E, Poblador M, Lancho. **Effects of training exercises for the development of strength and endurance in soccer.** *Journal of Strength and Conditioning Research.* 22(2); Pp 518-523. 2008.

26. Poliquin C. PICP Certification Level I-IV Internships and personal conversation. 2006-2012.

27. Schnieder, V, Arnold, B, Martin, K, Bell, D, Crocker, P. **Detraining Effects in College Football Players During the Competitive Season.** *Journal of Strength and Conditioning Research.* 12(1); Pp 42-45. 1998.

28. Siff M. **Recommended strength ratios: Part I.** *Fitness and Sports Review International.* 29(1); Pp 12-14. 1994,

29. Siff M. **Recommended strength ratios.** *Fitness and Sports Review International.* 29(2); Pp 78-80. 1994

30. Siff M. **How strenuous is that exercise.** *Fitness and Sports Review International.* 28(5-6); Pp 192-194. 1993.

31. Siff, M. **Autoregulating Progressive Resistance Exercise.** *Supertraining.* Pp259-262. Denver, Co 2004

32. Stone M. **Muscle conditioning and muscle injuries**. *Medicine and Science in Sports and Exercise.* 22(4); Pp 457-462. 1990,

33. Stone M, Sanborn K, Obryant H, Hartman M, Stone M, Proulx C, Ward B, Hruby J. **Maximum strength-power-performance relationships in collegiate throwers.** *Journal of Strength and Conditioning Research.* 17(4); Pp 739-745. 2003

34. Yessis, M. *Secrets of Soviet Sports Fitness and Training.* Collins Publishing. Ontario, 1987.

35. Zatsiorsky, V., Kreamer, W., **Training Residuals.** *Science and Practice of Strength Training.* Second Edition, Champaign Ill, Pp100-106, 2006.

36. Zatsiorsky, V. **Two Factor Theory (Fitness-Fatigue Theory).** *Science and Practice of Strength Training.* 2nd Ed. Pp12-15 Champaign Ill, 2006.

Chapter II

1. Cormie P, McCauliey G, Triplett N, Mcbride J. **Optimal loading for maximal power output during lower-body resistance exercises.** *Medicine and Science in Sports and Exercise.* 39(2); Pp 340-349. 2007.

2. Cormie P, McCauliey G, Mcbride J. **Power versus strength-power jump squat training: influence on the load-power relationship**. *Medicine and Science in Sports and Exercise.* 39(6); Pp 996-1003. 2007.

3. Folland J, Williams A. **The adaptations to strength training: morphological and neurological contributions to increased strength.** *Sports Medicine.* 37(2); Pp 145-168. 2007

4. Gabriel D, Kamen G, Frost G. **Neural adaptations to resistive exercise: mechanisms and recommendations for training practices.** *Sports Medicine.* 36(2); Pp 133-149. 2006

5. Poliquin C. PICP Level IV Certification Internship. 2010.

6. Schnieder, V, Arnold, B, Martin, K, Bell, D, Crocker, P. **Detraining Effects in College Football Players During the Competitive Season.** *Journal of Strength and Conditioning Research.* 12(1); Pp 42-45. 1998.

Chapter III

1. D'antona G, Lanfranconi F, Pellegrino M, Brocca L, Adami R, Rossi R, Moro G, Miotti D, Canepari M, Bottinelli R. **Skeletal muscle hypertrophy and structure and function of skeletal muscle fibres in male bodybuilders.** *The Journal of Physiology.* 570 (3); Pp 611-627. 2006.

2. Folland J, Williams A. **The adaptations to strength training: morphological and neurological contributions to increased strength.** *Sports Medicine.* 37(2); Pp 145-168. 2007

3. Gabriel D, Kamen G, Frost G. **Neural adaptations to resistive exercise: mechanisms and recommendations for training practices.** *Sports Medicine.* 36(2); Pp 133-149. 2006

4. Hakkinen K, Keskinen K. **Muscle Cross-Sectional Area and Voluntary Force Production Characteristics in Elite Strength and Endurance Trained Athletes and Sprinters.** *European Journal of Applied Physiology.* 59; Pp 215-220. 1989.

5. Schoenfeld B. **The mechanisms of muscle hypertrophy and their application to resistance training.** *Journal of Strength and Conditioning Research.* 24(10); Pp 2857-2872. 2010.

6. Schoenfeld B. **The mechanisms of muscle hypertrophy and their application to resistance training.** *Journal of Strength and Conditioning Research.* 24(10); Pp 2857-2872. 2010.

7. Tesch P. **Skeletal muscle adaptations consequent to long-term heavy resistance training.** *Medicine and Science in Sports and Exercise.* 20(5); Pp 132-134. 1988.

Chapter IV

1. Anderson A, Meador K, McClure L, Makrozahopoulos D, Brooks D, Mirka G. **A biomechanical analysis of anterior load carriage.** *Ergonomics.* 50(12); Pp 2104-2117. 2007.

2. Bartonietz , K. E. **Biomechanics of the snatch: toward a higher training efficiency.** *Journal of Strength and Conditioning* 18;Pp 24-31. 1996

3. Bissas A, Havenetidis K. **The use of various strength-power tests as predictors of sprint running performance.** *Journal of Sports Medicine and Physical Fitness.* 48(1); Pp 49-54. 2008.

4. Callaghan J, McGill S. **Muscle activity and low back loads under external shear and compressive loading.** *Spine.* 20(9); Pp 992-998. 1995.

5. Fry A, Kraemer W, Stone M, Warren B, Fleck S, Kearney J, Gordon S. **Endocrine responses to overreaching before and after 1 year of weightlifting.** *Canadian Journal of Applied Physiology.* 19(4); Pp 400-410. 1994.

6. Hamlyn N, Behm D, Young W. **Trunk muscle activation during dynamic weight-training exercises and isometric instability activities.** *Journal of Strength and Conditioning Research.* 21(4); Pp 1108-1112. 2007.

7. Hori N, Newton R, Andrews W, Kawamori N, McGuigan M, Nosaka K. **Does performance of hang power clean differentiate performance of jumping, sprinting, and changing of direction?** *Journal of Strength and Conditioning Research.* 22(2); Pp 412-418. 2008.

8. Mazzetti S, Douglass M, Yocum A, Harber M. **Effect of explosive versus slow contractions and exercise intensity on energy expenditure.** *Medicine and Science in Sports and Exercise.* 39(8); Pp 1291-1301. 2007.

9. McGill S, McDermott A, Fenwick C. **Comparison of different strongman events: trunk muscle activation and lumbar spine motion, load, and stiffness.** *Journal of Strength and Conditioning Research.* 23(4); Pp 1148-1161. 2009.

10. Mujika I, Santisteban J, Castagna C. **In-season effect of short term sprint and power training programs on elite junior soccer players.** *Journal of Strength and Conditioning Research.* 23(9); Pp 2581-2587. 2009.

11. Siff, M. *Supertraining.* Denver, Co. Pp 268. 2003.

12. Sleivert G, Taingahue M. **The relationship between maximal jump-squat power and sprint acceleration in athletes.** *European Journal of Applied Physiology.* 91(1); Pp 46-52. 2004.

13. Smirniotou A, Katsikas C, Paradisis G, Argeitaki P, Zacharogiannis E, Tziortzis S. **Strength-power parameters as predictors of sprinting performance.** *Journal of Sports Medicine and Physical Fitness.* 48(4); Pp 447-454. 2008.

14. Stone M, Sands W, Pierce K, Carlock J, Cardinale M, Newton R. **Relationship of maximum strength to weightlifting performance.** *Medicine and Science In Sports and Exercise.* 37(6); Pp 1037-1043. 2005.

15. 14.Tricoli V, Lamas L, Carnevale R, Ugrinowitsch C. **Short-term effects on lower-body functional power development: weightlifting vs. vertical jump training programs.** *Journal of Strength and Conditioning Research.* 19(2); Pp 433-437. 2005.

Chapter V

1. Anderson A, Meador K, McClure L, Makrozahopoulos D, Brooks D, Mirka G. **A biomechanical analysis of anterior load carriage.** *Ergonomics.* 50(12); Pp 2104-2117. 2007.

2. Hamlyn N, Behm D, Young W. **Trunk muscle activation during dynamic weight-training exercises and isometric instability activities.** *Journal of Strength and Conditioning Research.* 21(4); Pp 1108-1112. 2007.

3. Kurz T. *Science of Sports Training.* Stadion Publishing Company. Island Pond, VT. Pp 222-223. 1991.

4. McGill S, McDermott A, Fenwick C. **Comparison of different strongman events: trunk muscle activation and lumbar spine motion, load, and stiffness.** *Journal of Strength and Conditioning Research.* 23(4); Pp 1148-1161. 2009

Chapter VI

1. Blomstrand E, Eliasson J, Karlsson H, Kohnke R. **Branched-chain amino acids activate key enzymes in protein synthesis after physical exercise.** *The Journal of Nutrition.* 136(1); Pp 269-273. 2006.

2. Karlsson H, Nilsson P, Nilsson J, Chibalin A, Zierath J, Blomstrand E. **Branched-chain amino acids increase p70S6k phosphorylation in human skeletal muscle after resistance exercise.** *American Journal of Physiology, Endocrinology, and Metabolism.* 287(1); Pp E1-7. 2004.

3. Crayhon R. Nutrition Made Simple: A Comprehensive Guide to the Latest Findings in Optimal Nutrition. M. Evans and Company. 1996.

Chapter VII

1. Aggarwal B, Harikumar K. **Potential therapeutic effects of curcumin, the anti-inflammatory agent, against neurodegenerative, cardiovascular, pulmonary, metabolic, autoimmune and neoplastic diseases.** *International Journal of Biochemistry and Cell Biology.* 41(1); Pp 40-59. 2009.

2. Aggarwal B, Sundaram C, Malani N, Ichikawa H. **Curcumin: the Indian solid gold.** *Advances in Experimental Medicine and Biology.* 595; Pp 1-75. 2007.

3. Anto R, Mukhopadhvay A, Denning K, Aggarwal B. **Curcumin (diferuloylmethane) induces apoptosis through activation of caspase-8, BID cleavage and cytochrome c release: its suppression by ectopic expression of Bcl-2 and Bcl-xl.** *Carcinogenisis.* 23(1); Pp 143-150. 2002.

4. Beck T, Housh T, Johnson G, Schmidt R< Housh D, Coburn J, Malek M, Mielke M. **Effects of a protease supplement on eccentric exercise induced markers of delayed onset muscle soreness and muscle damage.** *Journal of Strength and Conditioning Research.* 21(3); Pp 661-667. 2007

5. Budoff, Je. **The Prevalence of Rotator Cuff Weakness in Patients with Injured Hands.** *The Journal of Hand Surgery.* 29(6); Pp 1154-1159. 2004.

6. Donath F, Mai I, Maurer A, Brockmoller J, Kuhn C, Friedrich G, Roots I. **Dose-related bioavailability of bromelain and trypsin after repeated oral administration.** *American Society for Clinical Pharmacology and Therapeutics.* 61; Pp 157. 1997.

7. Jurenka J. **Anti-inflammatory properties of curcumin, a major constituent of Curcuma longa: a review of preclinical and clinical research.** *Alternative Medicine Review.* 14(2); Pp 141-153. 2009.

8. Kolac C, Streichhan P, Lehr C. **Oral bioavailability of proteolytic enzymes.** *European Journal of Pharmaceutics and Biopharmaceutics.* 42 (4); Pp 222-232. 1996.

9. Maurer H. **Bromelain: Biochemistry, pharmacology and medical use.** *Cellular and Molecular Life Sciences.* 58(3); Pp 1234-1245. 2001.

10. Miller P, Bailey S, Barnes M, Derr S, Hall E. **The effects of protease supplementation on skeletal muscle function and DOMS following downhill running.** *Journal of Sports Sciences.* 22*4); Pp 365-372. 2004.

11. Ratamess N, Faigenbaum A, Mangine G, Hoffman J, Kang J. **Acute muscular strength assessment using free weight bars of different thickness.** *Journal of Strength and Conditioning Research.* 21(1); Pp 240-244. 2007.

12. Ravindran J, Prasad S, Aggarwal B. **Curcumin and cancer cells: how many ways can curry kill tumor cells selectively?** *AAPS J.* 11(3); Pp 495-510. 2009.

13. Yasuo, G, T Daisaku, M Nariyuki, S Jun'ya, O Toshihiko, M Masahiko, and M Yoshiyuki. **Relationship Between Grip Strength and Surgical Results in Rotator Cuff Tears.** *Shoulder Joint.* 29(3); Pp 559-562. 2005.

Chapter VIII

1. Esformes J, Cameron N, Bompouras T. **Postactivation potentiation following different modes of exercise.** *Journal of Strength and Conditioning Research.* 24(7); Pp 1911-1916. 2010.

2. Fletcher L, Jones B, **The Effect of Different Warm-up Stretch Protocols on 20 Meter Sprint Performance in Trained Rugby Union Players** *Journal of Strength and Conditioning Research.* 18(4); Pp 885-888. 2004.

3. Javorek, I. Personal Conversation. 2011.

4. Little T, Williams A, **Effects of Differential Stretching Protocols During Warm-up on High-Speed Capacities in Professional Soccer Players** *Journal of Strength and Conditioning Research.* 20(1); Pp 203-207. 2006.

5. Mcbride J, Nimphius S, Erickson T. **The acute effects of heavy-load squats and loaded countermovement jumps on sprint performance.** *The Journal of Strength and Conditioning Research.* 19(4); Pp 893-897. 2005.

6. Robbins, D.W. (2005). **Postactivation potentiation and its practical applicability: a brief review.** *Journal of Strength and Conditioning Research,* 19(2), 453-458.

7. Volek, J. Personal Conversation. 2012.

8. Young W, Behm D **Should Static Stretching Be Used during a Warm up for Strength and Power Activities?** *NSCA Journal.* 24(6); Pp 33-37. 2002.

Chapter IX

Football Programming

1. Biderman D. **11 Minutes of Action**. *Wall Street Journal.* 2010.

2. Swindler R. **Predicting 40-yard dash time in college football players.** *I.A.H.P.E.R.D. Journal.* 1999.

Soccer Programming

1. Bloomfield, J., Polman, R. O'Donoghue. **Physical demands of different positions in FA Premier League soccer.** *Journal of Sports Science and Medicine.* 6; Pp 63–70. 2007.

2. Spencer M., Bishop D., Dawson B., Goodman, C. **Physiological and metabolic responses of repeated sprint activities: Specific to field-based team sports.** *Sports Medicine.* 35; Pp 1025-1044. 2005.

Baseball Programming

1. Coleman, E, Dupler, T. **Changes in running speed in game situations during a season of Major League Baseball.** *JEPonline.* 7; Pp 89-93. 2004.

Hockey Programming

1. Bracko, M. **Time Motion Analysis of the Skating Characteristics of Professional Ice Hockey Players.** *Ph.D. Dissertation. Brigham Young University,Department of Physical Education.* 1992.

2. Twist P, Rhodes T. **A Physiological Analysis of Ice Hockey Positions.** *National Strength and Conditioning Association Journal.* 15(6); Pp 44-46. 1993.

Basketball Programming

1. Ben Abdelkrim N, Castagna C, Jabri I, Battikh T, El Fazaa S, El Ati J. **Activity profile and physiological requirements of junior elite basketball players in relation to aerobic-anaerobic fitness.** *Journal of Strength and Conditioning Research.* 24(9); Pp 2330-2342. 2010.

2. Ben Abdelkrim N, El Fazaa S, El Ati J. **Time-motion analysis and physiological data of elite under 19-year-old basketball players during competition.** *British Journal of Sports Medicine.* 41(2); Pp 69-75. 2007.

Field Hockey Programming

1. Spencer M., Bishop D., Dawson B., and Goodman, C. **Physiological and metabolic responses of repeated sprint activities: Specific to field-based team sports.** *Sports Medicine.* 35:Pp 1025-104.2005.

2. Spencer M, Lawrence S, Rechichi C, et al. **Time-motion analysis reduced when subsequent sprints are performed, sis of elite field-hockey: special reference to repeated-sprint activity.** *Journal of Sports Science.* 22; Pp 843-850. 2004.

Lacrosse Programming

1. Dintiman G, Ward B. *Sports Speed, (3),* Pp 14, 152.2003.
2. Schmidt MN, Gray P, Tyler S. **Selected fitness parameters of college female lacrosse players.** *Journal of Sports Medicine and Physical Fitness.* 21(3); Pp 282-290. 1981

3. Shaver LG. **Body composition, endurance capacity and strength of college lacrosse players.** *Journal of Sports Medicine and Physical Fitness.* 20(2); Pp 213-220.1980

Rugby Programming

1. Coughlan G, Green B, Pook P, Toolan E, O'Connor S. **Physical game demands in elite rugby union: a global positioning system analysis and possible implications for rehabilitation.** *Journal of Orthopedic and Sports Physical Therapy.* 41(8); Pp 600-605. 2011.

2. Cunniffe B, Proctor W, Baker J, Davies B. **An Evaluation of the Physiological Demands of Elite Rugby Union using Global Positioning System Tracking Software.** *Journal of Strength and Conditioning Research.* 23(4); Pp 1195-1203. 2009.

3. Roberts S, Trewartha G, Higgitt R, El-Abd J, Stokes K. **The physical demands of elite English rugby union.** *Journal of Sports Sciences.* 26(8); Pp 825-833. 2008.

Softball Programming

1. Axe M, Windley T, Snyder L. **Data based interval throwing programs for collegiate softball players.** *Journal of Athletic Training.* 37:2; Pp 194-203. 2002.

2. Flyger N, Button C, Rishiraj N. **The science of softball: implications for performance and injury prevention.** *Sports Medicine.* 36(9); Pp 797-816. 2006.

3. Messier S, Owen M. **Bat dynamics of female fast pitch softball batters.** *Research Quarterly for Exercise and Sport.* 55:2; Pp 141-145. 1984.

4. Werner S, Jones D, Guido J, Brunet M. **Kinematics and kinetics of elite windmill softball pitching.** *American Journal of Sports Medicine.* 34; Pp 597-603. 2006.

Tennis Programming

1. Bergeron M, Maresh C, Kraemer W, Abraham A, Conroy B, Gabaree C. **Tennis: a physiological profile during match play.** *International Journal of Sports Medicine.* 12(5); Pp 474-479. 1991.

2. Escamilla R, Andrews J. **Shoulder muscle recruitment patterns and related biomechanics during upper extremity sports.** *Sports Medicine (Auckland, NZ).* 39(7); Pp 569-590. 2009.

3. Fernandez J, Mendez-Villanueva A, Pluim B. *Intensity of tennis match play.* *British Journal of Sports Medicine.* 40; Pp 387-391. 2006.
4. Kovacs M. **Applied physiology of tennis performance.** *British Journal of Sports Medicine.* 40; Pp 381-386. 2005.

Volleyball Programming

1. Kraemer W., Hakkinen K. *Strength Training for Sport.* Pp 109 . Blackwell Sciences, 2002.

About The Author

With over 16 years of practical experience as a coach and educator, Jason Shea has earned a reputation as a strength coach and body composition specialist capable of training athletes and trainees at the highest levels. As the owner of APECS (www.apecs.com) and CrossFit Tri-Valley (www.crossfit-trivalley.com) Jason has earned the distinguished honor of being recognized as one of less than a dozen PICP Level IV International Strength Coaches in the U.S. His clientele has included professional, college, high school, and Olympic hopeful athletes as well as Fortune 500 business executives, SWAT Teams, military personnel, state and local firefighters, and more than 40 local high school, club, and college teams.

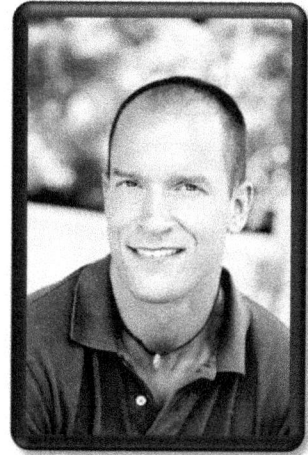

He has been strength coach to 2 High School Super Bowl Teams, 5 State Champion Lacrosse Teams, numerous State and New England Champion wrestlers and track athletes, Boston Globe Players of the year in Football, Volleyball, Wrestling, Lacrosse, and Soccer, over 25 High School and College league MVP's from all sports, College and high school league all-stars in nearly every sport, and league champion teams in high school sports including Football, Field Hockey, Soccer, Basketball, Hockey, Baseball, Field Hockey, Lacrosse, Wrestling, and Softball.

Jason holds a Bachelor's Degree in Exercise Science and a Master's in Human Movement. He has been certified through various organizations including the USAW, NASM, NSCA, ISSA, ACE, and PICP. Not one to rest on his laurels, Jason has traveled throughout the US and Europe to learn the most effective techniques in training, soft tissue, nutrition, and body composition taught by the Poliquin Strength Institute and PICP Certification Program.

Along with his role as Head Strength Coach at APECS and CrossFit Tri-Valley Jason is also the Massachusetts Statewide Health and Wellness Coordinator for the Municipal Police Training Committee. In this role he is responsible for academy certification and dissemination of continuing education for municipal police officers teaching at the Municipal Police Academies in Massachusetts.

The success of his business and clientele has led to current positions as Adjunct Professor in the Sport Fitness department at Dean College, consulting Strength Coach to the highly successful Dean College Football and Soccer Teams, Performance Director for the Speed and Power Academy at Franklin High School, Strength and Conditioning Coach to the nationally ranked Boston Irish Wolfhounds Rugby Team, columnist for the Metrowest Daily News, and the opportunity to co-author Law Enforcement articles with world renowned strength coach Charles Poliquin. He has also been a featured lecturer on strength and conditioning topics for various organizations including local colleges, corporation and high schools, Blue Chip Football Camps, and club teams in all sports.

Most important to Jason is the time he spends with his inspirations; son Ayden, daughter Bryn, and beautiful wife Wendy.

www.ingramcontent.com/pod-product-compliance
Lightning Source LLC
Chambersburg PA
CBHW081653270326
41933CB00017B/3154